Nutrition for Your Pregnancy
The University of Minnesota Guide

Nutrition
for
Your
Pregnancy

The University of Minnesota Guide

Judith E. Brown

University of Minnesota Press □ Minneapolis

RG
559
B74

Copyright ©1983 by the University of Minnesota.
All rights reserved.
Published by the University of Minnesota Press,
2037 University Avenue Southeast, Minneapolis, MN 55414
Printed in the United States of America.

Library of Congress in Publication Data

Brown, Judith E.
  Nutrition for your pregnancy.

  Bibliography: p.
  Includes index.
  1. Pregnancy—Nutritional aspects. I. Title.
RG559.B76 1983   618.2'4   82-21852
ISBN 0-8166-1151-3

The University of Minnesota
is an equal-opportunity
educator and employer.

This book is dedicated to Rita Evelyn Brown, the mother who taught me to eat right and the grandmother who showered our kids with love; and to Joe, Amanda, and Max, the three best parts of my life.

Contents

Foreword

Pregnant women have always accepted the importance of diet during pregnancy. Just how important diet is for mothers is finally being realized by health professionals. In the last ten years there has been a veritable explosion of books, pamphlets, and guides. In most cases information prepared by professionals for the general public was either too technical or too impersonal. At the other extreme, popular books prepared for the pregnant woman have tended to have little scientific credibility.

In this book, Judith Brown has fulfilled her intention of writing a guide that is readable, useful, accurate, and affordable. The tone throughout the book is upbeat and supportive. Essential topics are covered with sufficient detail to allow women to make informed choices. A noteworthy inclusion is the section on the need to stay physically fit.

This book, with its combination of impeccable accuracy, personal involvement in the problems of women, and emphasis on the positive, will be a major influence in helping women improve the course and outcome of their pregnancies.

Howard N. Jacobson, M.D.
Institute of Nutrition
University of North Carolina

Acknowledgments

We grow and eventually succeed on the shoulders of those who came before us. For the making of this book, there was a parade of people and shoulders. Agnes Higgins, former director of the Montreal Diet Dispensary, through her conviction and strength of character, helped produce for Canada and the United States two generations of "Blue Ribbon Babies." She encouraged me to dedicate myself to improving maternal and infant health through better nutrition.

Many of the opportunities I have had to study and teach in the area of maternal and child nutrition resulted from government initiatives in prenatal nutrition. The federal government has long recognized the importance of prenatal nutrition in promoting the birth of healthy babies to women who are at high risk of having too little to eat and who have poor health. These efforts are continued today by the federal office of Maternal and Child Health. I want to thank the following advocates for maternal and child health who have dedicated their careers to MCH and nutrition: Ms. Mary Egan, Ms. Marial Caldwell, and Dr. Howard Jacobson.

I thank the "friendly professionals" at the University of Minnesota Press for their steadfast encouragement and assistance.

My dream of writing this book could not have turned into reality without the help and encouragement given by my husband, Joe.

Preface

This book is for women who want to learn about the role nutrition plays in producing healthy babies. Because few women have access to a nutritionist before or during pregnancy, it's often hard for them to get reliable information about the relationship between their eating habits and the health of their unborn child. This situation needs to be changed. The bulk of evidence is perfectly clear: Good nutrition before and during pregnancy makes for healthy mothers and children; poor nutrition does not.

When a woman is pregnant or breast-feeding, her body has high nutritional demands. These demands must be met—and that takes a conscious effort. No "maternal instinct" exists that will draw a pregnant woman to a good diet and keep her from all things harmful. There is, however, a body of scientific knowledge about nutrition and pregnancy that a woman can use to help her make wise decisions about her diet during pregnancy.

Dietary advice has been given to pregnant women since ancient times. The specifics of that advice have changed dramatically over the centuries, not always for the better. Only in the past ten years have nutritional recommendations for pregnancy been based on careful scientific research rather than on clinical assumptions or folk-lore. Today we know more than ever about the advantages a mother gives her unborn child by eating well during pregnancy. We know that what and how much she eats, the amount of weight she gains, and her nutritional health coming into and leaving pregnancy can make a life-long difference in her child's health. My reason for writing this book is to share this scientific information with you so that you'll be able to give your own child a nutritional advantage at birth. For this information is of no use unless it reaches the people it can help — women like you who are either pregnant or planning a pregnancy.

Judith E. Brown

Nutrition for Your Pregnancy
The University of Minnesota Guide

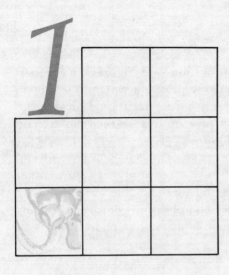

Giving Your Baby the "Nutritional Advantage"

Chris has just arrived. Her parents are ecstatic, speechless, wide-eyed, and exhausted. Chris is a beautiful baby. She is a thriving, pink, responsive, eight-pound, seven-ounce girl. During her first weeks at home, Chris nurses well, rarely fusses, and sleeps soundly. She is healthy, strong, and has a bright future.

Chris was born with an advantage—the nutritional advantage given to her by her mother—a gift she began receiving long before she was born.

Successful childbearing is influenced by many things, but none is as important as the health of the mother. And nothing affects a mother's health more than good nutrition. That's why you'll find a well-nourished, healthy mother with every well-nourished, healthy baby.

Today we are experiencing an explosion of new information about how children are affected by what their mothers eat before, during, and after pregnancy. Less than a decade ago, scientists believed that the nutrients an expectant mother took in with her food went first to her unborn child. They also believed that a mother could produce high-quality breastmilk no matter what she ate. And they believed "maternal instinct" would unconsciously direct an expectant mother to healthful foods.

We now know that all these assumptions are incorrect. Expectant mothers must consciously and actively pursue a wholesome diet to ensure that their unborn children receive the "nutritional advantage," a healthy start in life. Mothers can provide this for their children by following good, sound, nutritional knowledge.

It is worth the effort, for the nutritional advantage is a wonderful gift for mother and child alike. Study after study has shown that pregnant women who follow a healthy diet and gain an appropriate amount of weight experience fewer complications during pregnancy and at the time of delivery. And their babies are larger, healthier, and smarter than average.

In a sense, we are all what our mothers ate. The seeds of our health were planted by our mothers. How well our mothers cared for themselves and were cared for by others during their pregnancies influenced our health at birth. In turn, the babies you bear will reflect the nutritional advantage or disadvantage you inherited and built upon throughout your life.

When Planning a Pregnancy

Achieving the advantages that come with good nutrition can begin at anytime. But the sooner you get into good nutritional shape, the better. If you are planning a pregnancy, there are several steps you can take to become nutritionally ready. First, if you are overweight or underweight, you will want to adjust your weight to be as close to "normal" as possible. A chart listing average weights for various heights appears in Chapter 5 on page 40.

Second, you'll want to make sure that you are in good physical shape for pregnancy and that unhealthy aspects of your life-style, such as smoking and drinking, are tempered. The importance of these changes is discussed in Chapter 6.

Finally, you'll want to make sure you are eating a well-balanced diet. It's important to enter pregnancy with an adequate and varied supply of stored nutrients. This is especially true if you have been using contraceptive pills. Long-term use of the pill, coupled with poor diet, can increase your risk of becoming deficient in several vitamins, especially folic acid and vitamin B_6, during pregnancy. Fortunately, the extra need for these nutrients disappears within two to three months after you stop using the pill. That's why it has been recommended that women who have been on the pill wait at least three months before becoming pregnant. This time can be used to replenish the stores of vitamins and minerals that were used up at a higher-than-normal rate while you were taking the pill.

The best diet for pregnancy is a good diet that started before you became pregnant. How do you know if you're eating right? You can find out by taking a close look at your diet. Write down all the foods you ate yesterday, and the amount of each food, on the "My Diet" chart on page 6. Be sure to include snacks, beverages, and such items as sauces and spreads. If you are unsure about the amounts of food you eat, refer to food labels or measure your food and beverages with cups and tablespoons.

Now look at the "How Balanced Is My Diet before Pregnancy?" chart on page 7. It lists seven basic food groups. Match the foods and amounts on your list to these groups.

How did you do? Did you come up short in any of the food groups? If you did, you should fill in the gaps in your diet. Decide which foods you should and would eat more of, and which if any you should eat less of. Then, write down a daily food intake plan that includes a balanced diet that's right for you. A simple guide for planning balanced meals is given on pages 83-89. You can also use this guide for developing a shopping list that includes all the foods you need in your balanced diet.

What if you did not come up short in any of the groups? Congratulations! You are among the approximately twenty-five percent of Americans who have well-balanced diets.

Because most people's diets vary a lot from day to day, an analysis of several days of your diet will provide a more accurate accounting of the quality of your diet than one day will. Additional "My Diet" forms appear in the Appendix on pages 123-28.

If your diet isn't perfect, don't despair. That's what this book is about—learning what a good diet is, and what nutritional habits will allow you to eat right, gain the right amount of weight, and have the best chance to deliver and raise a healthy baby, one you've given the nutritional advantage!

My Diet

Time of Day	What I Ate and Drank	Date _____ Amount Consumed
Morning		
Mid-morning		
Noon		
Afternoon		
Evening		
Late evening		

How Balanced Is My Diet before Pregnancy?

Food Group	Size of Standard Serving	Number of Servings I Had	Minimum Recommended Number of Servings	Difference between my Servings and Number Recommended
1. Dairy products			2	
milk	1 cup			
yogurt	1 cup			
cheese	1 ounce			
cottage cheese	1 cup			
2. Meat and meat alternates			2	
meat	3 ounces			
fish	3 ounces			
poultry	3 ounces			
dried beans	1 cup			
eggs	2			
peanut butter	2 tbsp			
peanuts, other nuts	1/2 cup or 3 ounces			
3. Vitamin A vegetables and fruits			1	
broccoli	1/2 cup			
carrots	1/2 cup			
collards	1/2 cup			
green peppers	1/2 cup			
spinach	1/2 cup			
sweet potato	1/2 cup			
winter squash	1/2 cup			
papaya	1 cup			
cataloupe	1/4 melon			
plums	1 cup			
apricots	3			
4. Vitamin C fruits and vegetables			1	
cataloupe	1 cup or 1/4 melon			
oranges/orange juice	1 or 6 ounces			
grapefruit/juice	1 or 6 ounces			
tomatoes/juice	1 or 1 cup			
strawberries	2/3 cup			
watermelon	1/2 cup			
papaya	1/2 cup			
broccoli	1/2 cup			
raw cabbage	1 cup			
green pepper	1/2 cup			
brussel sprouts	1/2 cup			
5. Other fruits and vegetables			1	
banana	1			
apples/juice	1 or 6 ounces			
pears	1			

How Balanced Is My Diet before Pregnancy?—*Continued*

Food Group	Size of Standard Serving	Number of Servings I Had	Minimum Recommended Number of Servings	Difference between my Servings and Number Recommended
peaches	1			
grapes/juice	1/2 cup or 6 ounces			
potatoes	1 small or 1/2 cup			
corn	1/2 cup			
peas	1/2 cup			
beets	1/2 cup			
green beans	1/2 cup			
6. Breads and cereals			4	
bread	1 slice			
roll, biscuit, or muffin	1			
tortilla	1			
ready-to-eat cereal	3/4 cup			
pasta	3/4 cup			
rice	3/4 cup			
7. "Miscellaneous"			2 or more depending on calorie need	
Butter, margarine, oil	1 tsp			
salad dressing	2 tbsp			
sour cream	1 tbsp			
cream cheese	1 tbsp			
mayonnaise	2 tsp			
gravy	1 tbsp			

Planning a Balanced Menu before Pregnancy

Meal	Include at Least One Serving from Each of the Following Food Groups	Example
Breakfast	vitamin C fruit or vegetable	cantaloupe
	bread or cereal	whole-wheat toast with butter or margarine
	"miscellaneous"	
	meat or meat alternate	poached eggs
Lunch	bread or cereal	tuna salad sandwich
	meat or meat alternate	
	vitamin A vegetable or fruit	sliced tomatoes
	milk or milk product	milk
Supper	bread or cereal	spaghetti with meatballs
	meat or meat alternate	
	other vegetable or fruit	green beans, tossed salad
	milk or milk product	milk
Snack	other vegetable or fruit, or milk or milk product	apple or yogurt

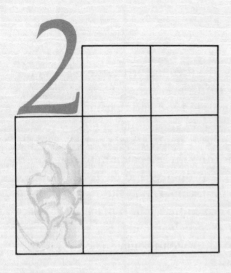

The ABC's
(and D's and E's)
of Nutrition

Lisa had just finished her morning-stretch exercises and was ready for breakfast. She poured herself a large glass of orange juice and a bowl of cereal. As she sat eating, her eye caught the side panel of the cereal box and the nutritional information listed there. Just yesterday she had heard a doctor talk on television about the importance of good nutrition during pregnancy. Because she was pregnant, she had listened carefully to what was said. Unfortunately, the talk had raised more questions than it had provided answers for. "What exactly is good nutrition?" she thought. "Which nutrients do I need for pregnancy? And what does all this information packed on the side panel of my cereal box mean?"

A well-balanced diet is one that includes daily servings from seven different food groups: dairy products, meat and meat alternatives, vitamin A vegetables and fruits, vitamin C fruits and vegetables, other fruits and vegetables, breads and cereals, and a "miscellaneous" group that includes fats and oils. A list of foods within these seven groups and their calorie values appears in the appendix on pages 90-93.

What's so magical about these seven groups? Why are all of them so important?

It has to do with sixty or so chemical substances needed by our bodies that are found in these groups of foods. We need adequate amounts of these substances, called *nutrients,* to grow, reproduce, and stay healthy. They enable us to do everything from blinking an eye and running a marathon to digesting food and fighting off disease. Without them, our cells—and we—would stop functioning.

A deficiency in any one nutrient can lead to serious health problems. For example, the body needs the nutrient calcium to clot blood, to make nerves and muscles function properly, and to develop bones. When it doesn't get enough calcium from food, the body steals it from its own bones. If that stolen calcium is not replaced, the body can get into trouble—though it may not become apparent for years. You could lose up to one-third of the calcium in your bones before the loss would show up on an X-ray.

Nor do nutrients function properly alone. Without vitamin D, for example, calcium cannot be absorbed from the intestines into the rest of the body.

It's important, therefore, that you feed your body—and that of your unborn child—all sixty nutrients. The only way you can do this is by eating a wide variety of foods because no one food (except breastmilk) has every nutrient in it.

Nutritionists have lumped nutrients into six general categories: protein, fats, carbohydrates, water, vitamins, and minerals. All are described in this chapter along with tips about the foods in which they can be found. Food sources of key nutrients are listed in detail in the appendix starting on page 93.

Protein

After water and possibly fats, protein is the most plentiful substance in the human body. It is the major building material for hair, skin, and nails. It also helps build the muscle tissue that holds the body's skeleton together. And it contributes to the formation of three important body chemicals: enzymes, which aid digestion and other body processes, antibodies, which fight off diseases and infection, and hormones, which regulate the body's chemistry.

Protein is especially needed when the body is rapidly creating new tissue. This, of course, is what happens during pregnancy as the fetus grows. After pregnancy, the mother's body continues to make new tissue—breastmilk.

So it's important that you get enough protein during pregnancy and afterward if you plan to breast-feed. You are, most likely, already consuming plenty of this nutrient. Most Americans eat much more protein than they actually need. About fourteen percent of the average American's calories comes from protein; the recommended figure is ten percent. Still, a significant portion of Americans—ten to fifteen percent—are *not* getting enough protein in their diets.

Protein varies in quality. The best comes from eggs, milk, cheese, meat, poultry, and fish. Some vegetables, especially soybeans, chickpeas, and peanuts are also good sources of protein.

Fats

Ounce for ounce, fats provide more energy—and, thus, more calories—than any other nutrient. Take a fatty food like butter, for example, and compare it to a high-carbohydrate food like an apple. An ounce of butter contains 200 calories; an ounce of apple, only 20 calories.

There are three distinct types of fats: saturated, polyunsaturated, and monounsaturated. Foods from animal sources, such as meat, eggs, milk, cheese, and butter, are high in saturated fats. Food from vegetable sources are usually high in either polyunsaturated fats (corn, sunflower, safflower, and corn oils) or monounsaturated fats (peanut and olive oils). Sometimes, however, foods from vegetable sources are high in saturated fats. This is true of chocolate, coconut, and avocados.

Saturated fats have been implicated in diseases of the heart and blood vessels among males. A diet overly rich in all three fats has been linked to breast cancer in women and colon cancer in men and women. Still, fats have their good points. They enable vitamins A, D, E, and K to be absorbed by the body. Linoleic acid, an important component of fats, keeps skin from becoming dry and scaly. And the body uses fat deposits to cushion and protect vital internal organs, such as the kidney.

You don't need to eliminate fats from your diet, but you should control the amount you eat. Here are a few easy ways to cut back on the fats you eat if you're worried about calories:

• Drink skim milk or two-percent milk instead of whole milk.
• Satisfy your protein requirement occasionally with beans or low-fat cheese instead of meat.
• Give up hot dogs, bologna, and other cold cuts of meat. They contain up to eighty percent fat.

- Cut off the fat from steaks and the skin from chicken and turkey meat before you eat them.
- Broil, bake, or boil your foods rather than fying them.

Carbohydrates

There are three types of carbohydrates: simple sugars, starches, and fiber. They serve as a major source of energy for your body. They are also frequently misunderstood.

Simple sugars exist naturally in fruits and other foods. These natural sources of sugar are healthy, for when we eat, say, a peach, we get fiber, vitamin A, vitamin C, potassium, and small amounts of niacin and iron as well as the sugar.

Most of the simple sugar we consume, however, is in the form of table sugar, honey, syrups, and candy. This sugar is added to foods, either by us in our own kitchens or by food manufacturers in their processing plants.

Simple sugar contains about fifty calories per tablespoon, but nothing else. No vitamins or minerals or protein. And the foods to which sugar is usually added—snack foods such as candy and pastries—tend to be low in vitamins and minerals and high in calories.

Despite sugar's negative characteristics, the average Americans continue to devour it at record rates—about 130 pounds each year. Fortunately, there is no convincing evidence that directly links sugar to heart attacks or blood-vessel disease. Nor, contrary to widespread opinion, does it cause diabetes. But when sugary foods are frequently substituted for healthier ones, health problems can result. Often, people who eat an abundance of sugary foods become overweight which, in turn, can lead to high blood pressure, diabetes, and other health problems, including tooth decay.

If you are concerned about the amount of sugar you eat, turn to fresh fruits instead of sweets. Identify which processed foods have added sugar. Finding sugar in processed foods isn't always easy. It involves reading food labels carefully. Look for these sugar pseudonyms: corn syrup, corn sweetener, honey, sorghum, dextrin, nutritive sweetener, and various words ending in "ose"—sucrose, lactose, levulose, maltose, dextrose, and fructose. They all mean sugar.

Contrary to general opinion, the second type of carbohydrates— starches, such as whole grains, potatoes, pastas, and dry beans—are generally low in calories and high in nutrients. Take one frequently maligned starchy food: the potato. A baked potato contains only 145 calories. Yet it also offers large amounts of vitamin C and potassium, and smaller amounts of niacin, vitamin B_1, folacin, vitamin B_6, phosphorus, magnesium, and iron. A nutritional bargain.

In addition, starchy foods like potatoes digest more slowly and release their energy into the body over a longer period of time than sugary foods. As a result, starchy foods satisfy your hunger better than sugars do.

Starchy foods are the major source of fiber in our diets. It passes through the body without being digested. This characteristic is precisely what makes fiber so important, for it helps keep food moving during digestion. Thus, eating high-fiber foods can help prevent constipation—a frequent complaint during pregnancy.

Unfortunately, much of the fiber is taken out of the foods we eat today. This is especially true of breads. The wheat berries from which most breads are made consist of three parts: endosperm, wheat germ, and bran. To make white flour and bread, only the endosperm is used; the wheat germ and bran are carted away. Whole wheat bread, on the other hand, is made from the *whole* wheat berry, including the wheat germ and bran. These latter two parts of the berry are what give whole wheat bread its light brown color—and most of its fiber. In addition, B vitamins, trace minerals (minerals required in very small amounts by the body), vitamin E, and some protein are lost when the bran and wheat germ are discarded. Enriching returns some of these nutrients to the bread, but not all. And it does not return the lost fiber.

A more healthful choice of breads, therefore, is one made from whole wheat or another whole grain (such as rye or buckwheat). Read food labels carefully. Don't be fooled by a bread that proclaims itself a "one hundred percent wheat bread." That's not the same as a one hundred percent *whole* wheat bread. And don't be fooled by a bread that looks brown. Bread manufacturers frequently add caramel coloring to white bread to make it look brown. Look at the ingredients listed on the wrapper. Make sure all the flour in the bread, or at least the first flour listed, is a *whole* grain flour.

Many other whole grain products, such as brown rice and whole wheat noodles, are available today in ordinary supermarkets. Ask your grocer where he or she has them stocked.

Water

Many people don't think of water as a nutrient. Yet it is the most important one there is. You can get along for days, even weeks, without food, but only a few days without water.

Water plays a major role in all processes of digestion. Most nutrients must dissolve in water so they may pass through the intestinal wall and into the bloodstream for use throughout the body. Water also carries waste out of the body and helps to regulate body temperature.

When you are pregnant or breast-feeding, you should drink at least ten glasses of fluid each day. Not all the water you drink need come directly from the kitchen tap. Fruit and vegetable juices, milk, and soups are also good sources of water.

Vitamins and Minerals

Thirteen vitamins exist in all. Four—A, D, E, and K—dissolve in fat rather than water. They enter the body with vegetable and fatty foods and are stored in body fat and in the liver until needed. The other nine vitamins—vitamin C and eight different B vitamins—are "water soluble." They dissolve in water and most cannot be stored in the body. An excess of these vitamins is soon excreted in the urine. You should include foods with these vitamins in your diet every day.

There are seven "major" minerals that are needed in relatively large amounts: calcium, phosphorus, chlorine, sodium, magnesium, potassium, and sulfur. The others, known as trace minerals, are required by the body in much smaller quantities. At least twenty of these trace minerals are needed for health, including iron, copper, and iodine.

The "My Daily Vitamin and Mineral Needs" chart on pages 15-17 lists key vitamins and minerals, the recommended daily allowance, their importance to the body, and the foods in which they can be found in large amounts. Are you getting enough of these foods? (For a more specific listing of foods and their nutrient contents, see pages 93-106 of the Appendix.)

A Special Word about Sodium (or Salt)

Sodium is a necessary nutrient, but most Americans consume much more sodium than they need. We get most of our sodium from

My Daily Vitamin and Mineral Needs

	Major Functions in Body	Best Food Sources	Recommended Daily Allowance for Women*		
			Nonpregnant	Pregnant	Breast-Feeding
		Vitamins			
Ascorbic acid	Promotes formation of blood vessels, skin, bones, tendons, and connective tissues; helps wounds heal.	Broccoli, brussel sprouts, orange juice, papaya, grapefruit juice, green peppers, strawberries.	60 mg. (about 2/3 cup of strawberries or 6 oz. of grapefruit juice.)	80 mg.	100 mg.
Vitamin B₁₂	Needed for the production of protein tissue and for normal red blood-cell development.	Liver, oysters, clams, fish, beef, lamb, eggs.	.003 mg. or 3 mcg. (About 6 oz. of roast or ground beef.)	.004 mg. or 4 mcg.	.004 mg. or 4 mcg.
Vitamin D	Helps body absorb and use calcium and phosphorus to make strong bones.	Vitamin D-fortified milk, fish liver oils; can also be produced in the body by exposing the skin to sunlight.	.005 mg. or 200 IU (About 2 cups of milk.)	.01 mg. or 400 IU.	.01 mg. or 400 IU.
Folacin	Helps body form protein tissues and develop normal red blood cells.	Leafy vegetables, asparagus, melons, orange juice, wheat germ, liver.	.4 mg. or 400 mcg. (about 3 cups of asparagus or spinach, 1 cantaloupe.)	.8 mg. or 800 mcg.	.5 mg. or 500 mcg.
Niacin (Vitamin B₃)	Helps convert food into energy; promotes a normal appetite; helps nerves function.	Liver, tuna, chicken, salmon, veal, peanuts, pork.	13 mg. (About 3 oz. of tuna or chicken.)	15 mg.	18 mg.
Pantothenic acid	Helps convert food into energy.	Liver, eggs, milk, dried beans, bananas.	7 mg. (About 3 oz. of liver.)	No recommendation available.	No recommendation available.
Pyridoxine (Vitamin B₆)	Helps form protein tissues, such as red blood cells, antibodies, and muscles.	Turnip greens, brussel sprouts, dried beans, liver, oysters, chicken, bananas, potatoes.	2 mg. (About 2 cups of dried beans.)	2.6 mg.	2.5 mg.

My Daily Vitamin and Mineral Needs—*Continued*

	Major Functions in Body	Best Food Sources	Recommended Daily Allowance for Women*		
			Nonpregnant	Pregnant	Breast-Feeding
Retinol (Vitamin A)	Helps form bones and teeth; maintains mucous membranes within the digestive tract; prevents night blindness.	Liver, carrots, spinach, sweet potatoes, collards, winter squash, broccoli.	.08 mg. or 800 mcg. RE (About 1/3 cup of carrots or 1 cup of broccoli.)	1 mg. or 1000 mcg. RE or 5000 IU.	1.2 mg. or 1200 mcg. RE or 6000 IU.
Riboflavin (Vitamin B$_2$)	Helps release food into energy; helps develop healthy skin, eyes, and nerves.	Liver, milk, yogurt, cheese, collards, winter squash, asparagus.	1.2 mg. (About 1.5 oz of liver or 3 cups of milk.)	1.5 mg.	1.7 mg.
Thiamin	Promotes normal appetite and digestion, and helps supply the body with energy.	Pork, green peas, collards lima beans, dried beans, rice, sunflower seeds.	1 mg. (About 4 oz. of pork or ½ cup of sunflower seeds.)	1.4 mg.	1.5 mg.
Tocopherol (Vitamin E)	Protects cells from destruction by strengthening the membrane that encloses them.	Vegetable oils, wheat germ, spinach, collards, nuts, dried beans.	8 mg. TE or 12 IU. (About 2 tbsp. of vegetable oil.)	10 mg. TE or 15 IU.	11 mg. TE or 16.5 IU.
Minerals					
Calcium	Helps build bones and teeth; helps transmit nerve impulses.	Milk, yogurt, collards, cheese, cabbage, spinach.	800 mg. or .8 g. (About 2½ cups of milk or 4 oz. of cheese.)	1200 mg. or 1.2 g.	1200 mg. or 1.2 g.
Iodine	Helps thyroid glands function properly.	Iodized salt, oysters, scallops, lobster, crab.	.15 mg. or 150 mcg. (About ½ tsp. iodized salt or 10 oz. of seafood.)	.175 mg. or 175 mcg.	.2 mg. or 200 mcg.

My Daily Vitamin and Mineral Needs—*Continued*

	Major Functions in Body	Best Food Sources	Recommended Daily Allowance for Women*		
			Nonpregnant	Pregnant	Breast-Feeding
Iron	Major component of hemoglobin, which carries oxygen, in the blood; fosters normal growth and appetite; promotes resistance to infection.	Prune juice, oysters, liver, lima beans, dried beans, beef.	18 mg. (About 3½ cups of dried beans or 6 oz. of liver.)	30-60 mg. (Iron supplement recommended.)	30-60 mg. (Iron supplement recommended.)
Magnesium	Helps supply energy to the body; builds protein tissues; promotes normal muscle actions.	Bran cereal, chick peas, soy beans, tofu, spinach clams, wheat germ, nuts.	300 mg. (About 11/3 cups of bran cereal or 1 cup of tofu.)	450 mg.	450 mg.
Phosphorus	Helps form bones and teeth; balances body fluid within cells.	Milk, yogurt, cheese, nuts, whole grain breads, peanuts, eggs, dried beans.	800 mg. or .8 g. (About 11/3 cups bran cereal or 2½ cups yogurt.)	1200 mg. or 1.2 g.	1200 mg. or 1.2 g.
Zinc	Promotes normal growth of tissues and bone; helps heal wounds; promotes normal sense of taste and smell.	Oysters, dried beans, crab, beef, veal, turkey, lamb.	15 mg. (About 2 oysters or 2 cups of dried beans.)	20 mg.	25 mg.

*When reading nutritional information you may find that the measurement units used for nutrients varies. To help you interpret these labels, several forms of measuring (RDAs) are included in this chart. Here is a key to these measurements:

g. (gram)
mg. (milligram)
mcg. (microgram)
IU (international unit): A measurement of the amount of a vitamin or mineral needed to produce a particular biological effect that has been agreed upon as an international standard.
RE (retinol equivalent): A modern system of measurement used to indicate the amount of retinol that a vitamin compound will yield after conversion to an active form in the body.
TE (tocopherol equivalent): A measure of the amount of tocopherol that a vitamin compound will yield after conversion to an active form in the body.

common salt, which is forty percent sodium and sixty percent chloride. Many of the processed foods and beverages we buy at the grocery store or at fast-food restaurants are highly salted. A can of prepared soup, for example, contains about one teaspoon of salt.

Sodium helps maintain proper fluid balance in the body. Excessive amounts, however, can cause too much fluid to be retained and can contribute to high blood pressure. Of course, other factors, such as obesity and stress, also play a role in the development of high blood pressure. But if people with high blood pressure reduce their sodium intake, their blood pressure usually falls.

Excessive consumption of salt by nonpregnant women and men, however, contributes to the development of fluid imbalance and hypertension. The situation differs for pregnancy. Salt intake has not been shown to be related to hypertension that develops *during* pregnancy. Salt restriction during pregnancy can be harmful to both mother and baby. And it is ineffective in treating hypertension that occurs during pregnancy.

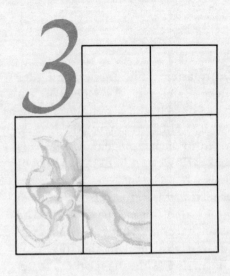

Eating Well During Your Pregnancy

Mary and John, both thirty-four years old, had been married since college twelve years before. John had quickly climbed the success ladder at his company and had just been promoted to Assistant Vice President of Marketing. Mary had worked as the manager of a women's fashion store. She left the job to slow down the pace of their lives when she found out she was pregnant. However, her life was still hectic because of the social schedule associated with John's new position. Both Mary and John were excited about the pregnancy. Mary's health was good and she thought this would carry her through pregnancy. Consequently, she paid little attention to her diet. Her primary concern was to keep her weight gain down so she could quickly get back her slender figure. She thought that a gain of twenty pounds would be right and that she shouldn't begin to "show" before five months. Periodically Mary cut down to 1000 calories a day to keep her gain low. Despite her physician's urging, Mary gained no weight after her seventh month of pregnancy when she had reached a twenty-pound gain and continued to consume a poorly balanced diet. Three weeks before her due date, Mary delivered a baby that was too small for its gestational age. After three days in the intensive-care nursery for management of low blood-sugar levels, the baby was transferred to the well-baby nursery and was followed closely by a pediatrician for the first six months of life.

We have all heard that during pregnancy you need to take special care with your diet because "you're eating for two." Actually you're eating for more like one and one-quarter. Still, the general idea behind the "eating for two" concept is correct. You need to eat enough during pregnancy to nourish yourself and a rapidly growing infant. And you must eat enough of the right foods. You could easily gain the thirty or so pounds you need to during pregnancy by eating mostly jelly beans and chocolate cake. However, that kind of weight gain does not make for healthy babies.

Here's why: It used to be believed that the fetus was at the head of the line when it came to getting nutrients from the mother. The fetus was viewed as a kind of parasite that took what it needed, even to the detriment of the mother. It was also thought that the fetus could get the nutrients it needed no matter what the mother ate, although where the fetus would get these nutrients was never fully explained.

Obviously, the fetus cannot get nutrients that the mother does not take in. And the fetus is denied full access to many nutrients that the mother has unless there is enough for them both. Most nutrients obtained from food will first go to supply the energy, vitamin and mineral storage needs of the mother. After the mother's needs have been satisfied, nurients then become available in sufficient quantities for placental and fetal growth.

Most nonpregnant women can lose ten to twenty percent of their body weight without endangering their lives. During pregnancy, however, such a weight loss seriously jeopardizes the health of both mother and baby. Rather than drawing upon maternal reserves to the point where the mother's health and ability to breast-feed are in jeopardy, fetal growth declines to spare the health of the mother—at the expense of the needs of the fetus.

A Good Diet for Pregnancy

If you follow the basic nutritional guidelines outlined in Chapter 2, you're well on your way to providing yourself and your unborn child with a healthy diet. You should make sure that during pregnancy your diet meets all of the following specific criteria:

• It should be well-balanced, supplying you and your unborn baby with all sixty key nutrients.

• It should provide enough calories to enable you to gain weight at an appropriate rate.

How Balanced Is My Diet for Pregnancy?

Food Group	Size of Standard Serving	Number of Servings I Had	Minimum Recommended Number of Servings	Difference between my Servings and Number Recommended
1. Dairy products			4	
milk	1 cup			
yogurt	1 cup			
cheese	1 1/2 ounce			
cottage cheese	1 cup			
2. Meat and meat alternates			2	
meat	3 ounces			
fish	3 ounces			
poultry	3 ounces			
dried beans	1 cup			
eggs	2			
peanut butter	4 tbsp			
peanuts, other nuts	1/2 cup or 3 ounces			
3. Vitamin A vegetables and fruits			1	
broccoli	1/2 cup			
carrots	1/2 cup			
collards	1/2 cup			
green peppers	1/2 cup			
spinach	1/2 cup			
sweet potato	1/2 cup			
winter squash	1/2 cup			
papaya	1 cup			
cataloupe	1/4 melon			
plums	1 cup			
apricots	3			
4. Vitamin C fruits and vegetables			1	
cataloupe	1 cup or 1/4 melon			
oranges/orange juice	1 or 6 ounces			
grapefruit/juice	1 or 6 ounces			
tomatoes/juice	1 or 1 cup			
strawberries	2/3 cup			
watermelon	1/2 cup			
papaya	1/2 cup			
broccoli	1/2 cup			
raw cabbage	1 cup			
green pepper	1/2 cup			
brussel sprouts	1/2 cup			
5. Other fruits and vegetables			2	
banana	1			
apples/juice	1 or 6 ounces			

How Balanced Is My Diet for Pregnancy?—*Continued*

Food Group	Size of Standard Serving	Number of Servings I Had	Minimum Recommended Number of Servings	Difference between my Servings and Number Recommended
pears	1			
peaches	1			
grapes/juice	1/2 cup or 6 ounces			
potatoes	1 small or 1/2 cup			
corn	1/2 cup			
peas	1/2 cup			
beets	1/2 cup			
green beans	1/2 cup			
6. Breads and cereals			4	
bread	1 slice			
roll, biscuit, or muffin	1			
tortilla	1			
ready-to-eat cereal	3/4 cup			
pasta	3/4 cup			
rice	3/4 cup			
7. "Miscellaneous"			2 or more depending on calorie need	
Butter, margarine, oil	1 tsp			
salad dressing	2 tbsp			
sour cream	1 tbsp			
cream cheese	1 tbsp			
mayonnaise	2 tsp			
gravy	1 tbsp			

• It should contain an adequate amount of high fiber foods.
• It should include ten cups of fluids each day.
• It should contain salt "to taste."
• It should limit or, better yet, exclude foods that contain caffeine or saccharin. It should exclude alcohol.
• And it should be tasty! You should enjoy the foods you eat.

During pregnancy you should periodically complete the "How Balanced Is My Diet" chart given on pages 21 and 22. Follow the same instructions that were given on pages 7 and 8 in Chapter 1.

Getting Started: In the Kitchen

Eating a balanced diet during pregnancy begins with planning nutritious and tasty menus. Fortunately, many good cookbooks are available offering recipes that are both delicious and healthful. Many of the newer cookbooks also stress recipes that are easy to prepare — a welcome feature during pregnancy when you may not feel like spending hours in the kitchen.

Listed below are a few of the better cookbooks. You should be able to find these books in your local library or bookstore. Or you can order them directly from their publishers.

Keep It Simple, 30-Minute Meals from Scratch
Burros, Marian, 1981. From William Morrow and Co., Inc., New York, NY. 300 pages.

This book is a treasure for pregnant women who find themselves too tired to cook in the evenings. All of the meals can be prepared within thirty minutes. They are also very healthy and well balanced, although some of the vegetarian meals may be a little low in calories. As bonuses, the book offers a short course in understanding exactly what goes into the foods you buy in the supermarket and some easy and inexpensive recipes for making "convenience" foods.

Recipes for a Small Planet
Ewald, E. B., 1973. From Ballantine Books, New York, NY. 356 pages.

This is a sequel to the best-selling *Diet for a Small Planet* by Frances Moore Lappe. Its discussion of how to combine certain foods to obtain complete protein dishes is a particularly useful guide for vegetarian meal planning. Each of its recipes is also analyzed for protein content.

The Family Health Cookbook
White, A. and the Society for Nutrition Education, 1980. From David McKay Co., Orangeburg, NY. 284 pages.

This cookbook provides a good deal of information about the principles of nutrition. Its recipes are all healthy and tasty, and should provide your family with more than a few favorites.

The American Diabetic Association Family Cookbook
The American Diabetes Association, 1980. From Prentice-Hall, Inc., Englewood Cliffs, NJ. 391 pages.

Although this book highlights recipes that meet the dietary needs of people with diabetes, it can be used and enjoyed by everyone. Topics include exercise and weight control, the basics of good nutrition, guidelines for eating out and brown-bagging, and easy-to-eat foods when one is ill.

Cooking to Stay in SHAPE
Franz, M. and Hedding, B., 1981. From SHAPE, 4959 Excelsior Blvd., Minneapolis, MN. 50 pages.
This cookbook was prepared as part of a wellness program. Its recipes are aimed at reducing the fat, sugar, and salt content of the average American's diet.

The Athlete's Kitchen
Clark, N., 1981. From CBI Publishing Co., Boston, MA. 284 pages.
This is a "how to" book aimed at helping athletes improve their daily training diet. Its recipes are nutritious as well as easy and quick to prepare.

Lean Cuisine
Gibbons, B., 1979. From Harper & Row, New York, NY. 50 pages.
This book provides a collection of delicious low-calorie recipes as well as helpful shopping and meal-planning tips.

American Heart Association Cookbook
Eshelman, R., 1979. From David McKay Co., Orangeburg, NY. 519 pages.
The recipes in this cookbook are provided for people who are trying to reduce their intake of saturated fat and cholesterol. It includes a chart of the fat and cholesterol content of foods. Some of its recipes, however, are high in salt and sugar. When following the recipes, you may want to use less of these two ingredients.

Laurel's Kitchen
Robertson, L., 1976. Nilgiri Press, Petaluma, CA. 641 pages.
A great book for anyone interested in vegetarian foods. It includes tasty, low-fat recipes and menus, and is especially helpful for people who want to "get back to the basics."

Getting the Most Out of Your Food

Many nutrients are lost during the processing, storage, and preparation of food. Prolonged storage, exposure to heat, or exposure to water during cooking can quickly reduce the value of fresh fruits and vegetables, especially those rich in the water-soluble vitamins (vitamin C and the B vitamins).

Vitamin C is the most fragile vitamin. This is especially true of the vitamin C found in non-acidic vegetables, such as broccoli, brussels sprouts, collard greens, and cauliflower. When these foods or their juices are cooked and then stored at room temperature for several hours, they rapidly lose their vitamin C. If you're eating these fruits and vegetables primarily for this vitamin, store them in a cool place and eat them raw or right after they are cooked.

The vitamin C found in acidic fruits, such as oranges, grapefruits, cranberries, and tomatoes, is much more stable. The acid medium partially protects the vitamin C from destruction, even during heating. It's still wise, however, to store these foods and their juices in a cool place and in air-tight containers.

The vitamin C that food manufacturers often add to non-acidic juices, such as apple juice or grape juice, or to artificially flavored drinks is *not* stable. It, too, disappears quickly once the juices or drinks are opened and exposed to light, air, and room temperature. So, if it's vitamin C you want from your juices, turn to the "real" things—orange, grapefruit, cranberry, and tomato juice.

Here are some tips to help you make sure you're getting the most nutrients out of the foods you eat:

- Serve fresh fruits and vegetables.
- Eat vegetables raw whenever possible. When you cook them, use only a small amount of water or, better yet, steam them. Then use the cooking water to make a soup or sauce. Don't overcook vegetables; they should be slightly crunchy when served.
- Avoid storing cooked vegetables. Prepare only enough for each meal and eat them right after they're cooked.
- Store foods and juices in air-tight containers in the refrigerator.

If You're a Vegetarian

You can be a vegetarian and still follow a nutritious, well-balanced diet during pregnancy. This is especially true if you are a lacto-ovo vegetarian (one who eats milk products and eggs). Just be sure you consider the following points when planning your diet:

- Because you are not eating meat or fish, you need other high-quality sources of protein. As a lacto-ovo vegetarian, you can find these meat substitutes in eggs, cheese, milk, and milk products. Include in your diet four servings from this group daily.

• Eliminating meat from your diet may result in a lower intake of iron. So make sure you're getting enough iron-rich foods. (See "My Daily Vitamin and Mineral Needs" chart on pages 15-17.)

If you are a vegan (a vegetarian who avoids all animal products), you must take added care in planning your diet. In fact, it is recommended that you consult a dietitian or nutritionist during your pregnancy for the following reasons:

• Many plant foods are low in calories. You must make sure you are eating enough food to enable you to gain weight during your pregnancy at an appropriate rate.

• Plant foods do not contain vitamin B_{12}. Your diet should include a vitamin B_{12} supplement.

• Most plant proteins are deficient in one or more of the eight essential amino acids. Without the presence of all eight amino acids, plant protein cannot be used by your body to build tissues. As a vegan, you must make sure you eat vegetables in combinations that provide all eight essential amino acids. Such combinations include:

rice and legumes
corn and legumes
whole wheat and legumes
soybeans and rice and whole wheat
sesame and dried beans
peanuts and sesame and soybeans
sesame and soybeans and whole wheat
peanuts and sunflower seeds

(Legumes are dried peas and beans of all types, including lentils and soy, pinto, garbanzo, navy, and lima beans.)

If You're a Teen-ager

Teen-age women have even more to gain from a good diet during pregnancy than older women—and more to lose from a poor one. That's because, as a group, teen-age women are more likely to develop health problems during pregnancy. Much, of course, depends on a young woman's life-style during her pregnancy—whether she gets enough exercise, for example, or uses drugs or alcohol—and how soon and how regularly she receives health care. But a lot also depends on her diet.

Teens with the highest risk of developing health problems during pregnancy are those who haven't yet finished growing. Most teen-agers complete their growth by the age of sixteen, or roughly four years after menstruation starts.

If you become pregnant before you have completely grown, you have a greater chance of delivering a premature or undersized baby. You also have a greater likelihood of developing preeclampsia or a nutritional anemia during your pregnancy. These two conditions present health threats to both you and your unborn baby. Preeclampsia is a pregnancy disorder that primarily affects the kidney and the circulatory system. Its cause is unknown, but its symptoms include high blood pressure, swelling of the ankles, hands, and feet, and protein in the urine. The advanced stages of preeclampsia can lead to convulsions and coma. Nutritional anemia is a blood disorder characterized by a shortage of nutrients needed to build red blood cells. It causes tiredness, poor appetite, and frequent illnesses. Babies born to anemic women have a high risk of becoming anemic themselves during their first year of life.

So if you're a pregnant teen-ager, it's especially important that you get all the nutrients you need. You must be extra picky about your food choices. Look again at the "How Balanced Is My Diet" chart on pages 21-22. You'll need to make some changes on it. Substitute the following recommended number of servings for those that appear in column 4 of the chart:

Dairy products	5 servings
Meat and meat alternatives	3 servings
Vitamin A vegetables	1 serving (same as on chart)
Vitamin C fruits and vegetables	2 servings
Other fruits and vegetables	1 serving (same as on chart)
Breads and cereals	5 servings

If you're like most busy teen-agers, snacks are probably an important part of your diet. In fact, most teen-agers eat about one-fourth of their food between meals. You don't have to stop snacking while you're pregnant, but you should choose as your snacks nutritious foods rather than "junky" ones. Both you and your unborn baby will need the nutrients these healthful snacks can provide.

Here's a list of snacks that are naturally delicious, quick-to-get, and rich in nutrients:

Nuts and seeds
Hard-boiled eggs
Raisins
Fruits (fresh, dried, or canned in natural or light syrups)
Crackers with peanut butter or cheese
Fruit and vegetables juices
Salads
Soups
Yogurt
Milk

Women with Extra Nutrient Needs

Teen-agers aren't the only pregnant women with extra nutrient needs. If, because of illness or poor diet, you enter pregnancy underweight or undernourished, you'll also need more nutrients than the average pregnant woman. This is especially true if you were using contraceptive pills until shortly before you became pregnant (see Chapter 1). Women who experience psychological stress during pregnancy—especially severe stress, such as from a divorce or the loss of a loved one—also have a higher nutrient requirement. For unknown reasons the body demands more nutrients during times of stress—and that can leave fewer nutrients for the unborn baby.

If you fit into one of these extra-need categories, you must make doubly sure that your diet is well balanced so that both you and your baby receive enough nutrients. Refer often to the "My Daily Vitamin and Mineral Needs" chart on pages 15-17.

Do You Need a Vitamin and Mineral Supplement?

Women who fall into the categories described above may benefit from taking a multi-vitamin and mineral supplement *while* they are improving their diet. The supplement can help speed up the recovery process. But it is only a short-term answer. Supplements should never be taken in place of a good diet, and they should be selected and monitored carefully.

For most women only two nutrients, iron and folic acid, are recommended in supplement form during pregnancy. These two nutrients have been singled out because anemia can occur if they are missing from the diet. Except for these supplements, taking a vitamin and mineral pill during pregnancy does not appear to be necessary for healthy women. During recent years at least fifteen studies have been conducted to see if pregnant women benefit from taking a multi-vitamin and mineral supplement, the kind that contains a hodge-podge of different vitamins and minerals. None of these studies found that the supplements were especially beneficial. The quality and quantity of a pregnant women's diet is much more closely related to the health of her newborn baby than whether or not she took a multi-vitamin and mineral pill during pregnancy.

In fact, taking a multi-vitamin and mineral supplement can create a health hazard for both you and your unborn baby. In some cases, it can upset the delicate balance of the various nutrients in your body. One commonly prescribed prenatal multi-vitamin and mineral pill, for example, contains no iron and from twenty-two to 600 percent of the Recommended Dietary Allowance (RDA) levels for fourteen other vitamins and minerals. Taking such a pill can lull you into believing that you are meeting your nutrient needs when, in truth, you may not be receiving some of the needed vitamins and minerals and dangerous overdoses of others.

Large doses of certain vitamins and minerals can be particularly health-threatening. High doses of vitamin A, vitamin D, and zinc, for example, can be poisonous to your unborn baby. In addition, vitamin C deficiency has occurred in very young infants whose mothers took large doses of vitamin C (one or more grams a day) during pregnancy. When a fetus receives a large amount of vitamin C, it rapidly excretes the excess. It soon gets so accustomed to excreting vitamin C that it continues to do so after it is born, even though it no longer receives an excess supply of the vitamin.

Unless you have a specific vitamin or mineral deficiency that has been verified through a blood test, any supplement you take should be close to the RDA levels. The "My Daily Vitamin and Mineral Needs" chart on pages 15-17 gives RDA's for nonpregnant, pregnant, and breast-feeding women. Another chart on pages 30-32 lists the possible symptoms of consuming too few or too many of certain vitamins and minerals. Make sure that any vitamin or mineral supplement you are taking contains amounts well below the unsafe levels reported on the chart.

Health Problems Resulting from Consuming Too Few or Too Many Vitamins and Minerals

Eating an unbalanced diet can result in the vitamin and mineral deficiency problems listed below. However, only in very, very rare instances—such as eating too much polar-bear liver, which contains extremely high levels of vitamin A—can you eat your way into the toxicity problems described below. These problems almost always stem from taking too high doses of vitamin and mineral supplements.

Also, remember that many of the symptoms listed below can be caused by illnesses not related to too few or too many vitamins and minerals in the diet. If you are experiencing these symptoms, consult your physician.

	Symptoms of Deficiency	Symptoms of Toxicity	Unsafe Daily Levels
		Vitamins	
Ascorbic acid (Vitamin C)	Dry, itchy skin; loss of hair; small hemorrhages (bleeding) at base of body hair; fatigue; swollen and bleeding gums; tender mouth; pain in joints.	Diarrhea; nausea. Infants may develop vitamin C deficiency if large doses of vitamin C were taken during pregnancy.	1000 mg. or 1 g.
Vitamin B_{12}	Sore tongue; weakness; loss of weight; apathy; nervous system disorders; anemia.	None reported.	None reported.
Biotin	Sleeplessness; muscle pain; loss of appetite; nausea; fatigue; depression; dermatitis.	None reported.	None reported.
Vitamin D	Retarded growth; weak bones; muscle weakness; listlessness.	Nausea; loss of appetite irritability; mental retardation; kidney damage.	.025 mg. or 25 mcg. or 1000 IU.
Folacin (Folic acid)	Smooth, red tongue; diarrhea; anemia; fatigue.	Excessive folacin may mask certain symptoms of pernicious anemia owing to a vitamin B_{12} deficiency.	None reported.
Vitamin K	Blood fails to clot or clots slowly; body bruises easily.	Synthetic vitamin K (menadione) has produced skin, hair, and respiratory tract irritation. Natural forms of vitamin K do not produce toxic symptoms.	None reported.
Niacin	Loss of appetite and weight; anemia; weakness; irritability; loss of sense of balance; sore mouth and tongue.	Flushing of skin; red rash on skin; headache; nausea; rapid heart beat.	2000 mg. or 2 g.

Health Problems Resulting From Consuming Too Few
or Too Many Vitamins and Minerals—*Continued*

	Symptoms of Deficiency	Symptoms of Toxicity	Unsafe Daily Levels
Pyridoxine (Vitamin B$_6$)	Greasy dermatitis around eyes, in the eyebrows, and at the corners of the mouth; dizziness; nausea; weight loss; kidney stones; anemia.	May produce liver disease.	1500 mg. or 1.5 g.
Retinol (Vitamin A)	Retarded growth; lack of ability to see well in dim light; dry and scay skin; diarrhea; intestinal infection.	Nausea; irritability; blurred vision; growth retardation; enlargement of spleen and liver; loss of hair.	2 mg. or 2000 mcg. RE or 10,000 IU.
Riboflavin (Vitamin B$_2$)	Retarded growth; anemia; scaly, greasy dermatitis around face and ears; sore throat and mouth; cracks at corners of mouth; lips redden and become sore; dim vision; burning sensation in eyes.	None reported.	None reported.
Thiamin (Vitamin B$_1$)	Retarded growth; loss of appetite and weight; fatigue; constipation; muscle cramps; numbness or tingling in toes and feet; mental confusion; apathy; disturbances in heart function.	Infants may develop a thiamin deficiency if large doses of thiamin were taken during pregnancy.	None reported.
Tocopherol (Vitamin E)	Anemia in adults, but only in very rare cases. In premature and low birth-weight babies, anemia from this deficiency is not as rare.	Anemia.	200 mg. TE or 300 IU.

Minerals			
Calcium	Retarded growth; weak bones and teeth; malformation of bones.	Calcium deposits in body organs and tissues.	200 mg. or 2 g.
Copper	Hemorrhage (bleeding); retarded growth; anemia.	Nausea; vomiting; low blood levels of vitamin A.	20 mg.
Fluoride	Tooth decay; growth retardation.	Discoloration of teeth; deformed teeth.	20 mg.
Iron	Loss of appetite; increased susceptibility to infection; fatigue; pale skin; anemia.	Gastrointestinal upsets (diarrhea, constipation). High intake from supplements can cause serious illness and death in children.	200 mg.

Health Problems Resulting From Consuming Too Few
or Too Many Vitamins and Minerals—*Continued*

	Symptoms of Deficiency	Symptoms of Toxicity	Unsafe Daily Levels
Selenium	None reported.	Discoloration of teeth; hair loss.	200 mg.
Zinc	Retarded growth and development; reproductive failures; abnormal glucose tolerance; loss of sense of taste; low birth-weight infants. It may also cause birth defects.	Fever; nausea; vomiting; diarrhea.	30 mg.
Other minerals	Weakness; disturbances in acid-base balance of body fluids; dehydration; and others.	All minerals are toxic when taken in excessive amounts.	Twice the RDA levels (see pages 15-17)

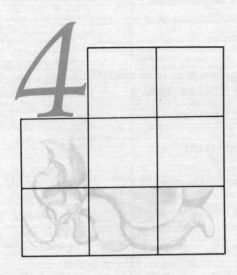

How Do Diet
and Weight Gain
Affect You
and Your Baby?

Evelyn is expecting her fifth child any day. She has had three living children and two miscarriages. One of her children died at 5 months of age from an infection. This pregnancy was managed like the others. Up until her eighth month of pregnancy, Evelyn was allowed to gain fifteen pounds. Then, she went on a low calorie, low carbohydrate, low fluid, and high protein diet for the rest of pregnancy. Evelyn's total weight gain was fourteen pounds. She will deliver a five-pound boy at thirty-eight weeks gestation. After a two-week rest, Evelyn will be allowed to get up, slowly, and walk around. Her son will grow poorly and will frequently be sick, as her other children were. She will feel fortunate that all but one of her children has survived childhood.

This story wouldn't have been unusual sixty years ago. Diets and weight gain then were often strictly controlled, usually to the detriment of the health of both mother and child.

What we now know about the benefits of optimum nutrition for pregnant women and children has taken an enormously long time to discover. Through the years, recommendations for "optimal" diets and weight gain have varied widely. Until recently, the health problems that resulted from improper advice rarely stood in the way of giving it. Nor did the positive health results from sound advice stand in the way of disregarding it. But now we know better—or, at least, we should.

The Old Myths

The general dietary advice offered pregnant women from Biblical times through the seventeenth century fostered good health for mothers and children alike. In *A Directory for Midwives*, first published in 1651 by the British astrologer and pharmacist Nicholas Culpeper, women were counseled that "when the child is bigger, let his diet be more, for it is better for women with child to eat too much than too little lest her child should want nourishment." (p. 120). The emphasis on fulfilling the baby's need for nourishment was also reflected in the belief during Culpeper's time that labor was brought on by the mother's inability to supply the baby with enough nourishment. When the baby needed more food, he or she would come out and get it!

This liberal approach to weight gain during pregnancy ended during the late eighteenth century. In 1788, James Lucas, a British surgeon, devised a special diet to help prevent the birth of babies too large to fit through abnormally small pelvises. Many women of Lucas's time had small pelvises because of vitamin D deficiencies suffered during childhood. Forced to work from dawn to dusk in the new factories of the industrial revolution, their bodies were seldom exposed to sunlight and, therefore, could not manufacture enough vitamin D for their growing bones. Nor did they have the modern advantage of vitamin D-fortified milk.

Lucas suggested that women with small pelvises be kept on a semi-starvation diet toward the end of their pregnancies to limit their unborn babies' growth. This may have been wise counsel in those pre-cesarean section days when women with very small pelvises frequently died during childbirth. Unfortunately, however, the use of the semi-starvation diet became a widely accepted practice. Many women with perfectly adequate pelvises were subjected to the Lucas diet, and their infants' size and health were compromised because of it.

This misguided belief that weight gain should be kept to a minimum during pregnancy resurfaced many times during the next two centuries. As late as the 1940s, doctors put their pregnant patients on unhealthy weight-restricting diets. A total weight gain of fifteen pounds was considered desirable; if a woman gained more than twenty pounds she was subjected to a strict and vigorous diet. During this era, the prescription and use of diet pills (amphetamines), water pills (diuretics), and low-calorie diets were common practice. The use of saccharin as a substitute for sugar was also encouraged. "Whenever saccharin can be substituted for one level teaspoon of sugar," advises *Expectant Motherhood*, a popular 1940s book for pregnant women, "twenty calories are deleted thereby—and every little bit helps." Salt restriction was similarly routine.

Pregnant women during the 1940s must have spent most of their time talking themselves out of their hunger and satisfying their sweet tooth with an artificial sweetener that is no longer recommended for pregnancy because of potential cancer risks.

The New Facts

The first study of the influence of a mother's diet on the health of her baby was performed in England in 1916. The study found that babies born to malnourished women were more frequently premature and were smaller than expected based on length of pregnancy. More of the babies born to poorly nourished mothers died than those born to women who were well nourished.

Almost three decades later, during World War II, additional studies were conducted in the Soviet Union, Holland, and England which added greatly to our understanding of nutrition and pregnancy. The war created conditions of famine in each of these three countries. Yet the impact of food shortages on the health of mothers and infants differed from country to country.

Women in the Soviet Union's Leningrad, where poor diets and hardship had existed before the war, were especially hard hit by the food shortages. Many women failed to conceive or lost their babies very early in pregnancy. More than forty percent of the babies born during the Leningrad famine were premature, and twice as many infants died during the first year of life.

The wartime food shortages that occurred in Holland left pregnant women with a daily average of 1000 calories and forty grams of protein, about the same level as women in Leningrad. But there was an important difference between the women in Holland and those in

Leningrad. Dutch women were generally well nourished before the war. As a result, fewer women in Holland were able to conceive and babies were smaller at birth than before the wartime food shortages. But the decreases in infant birth weights were not nearly as great as those in Leningrad. Being well nourished before pregnancy had helped to avoid the disastrous effects of long-term malnutrition seen in Leningrad.

In England pregnant women during the war received extra food rations. Because these special rations emphasized foods that helped meet the nutrient needs of pregnant women, the diets of these women actually improved. Babies born during the period of rationing weighed more at birth, and there were fewer cases of stillbirths, birth defects, and infant deaths.

These three World War II studies provide striking evidence of how eating well before and during pregnancy can help ensure the birth of a healthy newborn.

Right after the war, researchers at Harvard University uncovered more evidence that the adequacy or inadequacy of a woman's diet during pregnancy influences her newborn's birth weight, length, and general health. The Harvard researchers also discovered, as many have since, that how much a baby weighs at birth depends primarily on how much weight the mother gained during pregnancy and what she weighed before pregnancy. Healthy women who gain fifteen pounds during pregnancy will deliver, on the average, babies that weigh seven pounds. A gain of twenty-four pounds is associated with birth weights of seven pounds, six ounces. When thirty pounds are gained, babies tend to weigh eight pounds, one ounce at birth.

Today, the average birth weight of a baby born in the United States is about seven pounds, six ounces. Infant illness, disabilities, and death rates are lowest, however, for babies who weigh between *seven pounds, fourteen ounces and nine pounds*. So it is clear that the average birth weight of babies born in the United States is too low. Scientists predict that we would have healthier infants if the average birth weight would rise.

The birth weight of an infant is closely related to the child's future health and development. Studies in Sweden, Norway, and Finland have revealed that women in those countries give birth to babies with higher average weights than American babies. And the percentage of low-weight babies (those who weigh less than five pounds, eight ounces) born in those Scandinavian countries is about four percent, or nearly one-half that of the United States. As a result, Scandinavian infants are bigger, healthier, and fewer die during their first year of life.

Similar results were found in a large study funded by the National Institute of Health in this country. Babies born with above average birth weights (seven pounds, six ounces or more), concluded the study, have fewer diseases and are generally healthier than babies born at or below average weight. Weight at birth has also been associated with later intelligence scores. In a Detroit study, children in the highest average birth-weight group had the highest average IQ test scores; those with the lowest birth weights had significantly lower scores.

Although bigger than average babies tend to do better, extremely large babies do not. Babies with birth weights of more than ten pounds present slightly more than an average number of problems during labor and delivery. One such problem is shoulder dystocia, the large shoulders of the baby getting caught on the mother's pelvic bone during delivery. (The birth of babies weighing more than ten pounds, by the way, has not been found to be related to high weight gains during pregnancy.) It is, however, associated with obesity before pregnancy, poorly controlled diabetes during pregnancy, a pregnancy lasting longer than forty-two weeks, a family history of large newborns, and the position of the mother during labor. Shoulder dystocia is more likely to occur if you are lying on your back during delivery.)

Recent studies have also indicated that how much a baby weighs during the different stages of pregnancy makes a critical difference in his or her health. A baby born weighing six pounds, eight ounces after eight months of pregnancy will likely experience fewer health complications than a baby who weighs that much after nine months of pregnancy. Consequently, how much a baby weighs for his or her gestational age (length of pregnancy) is a more accurate indicator of growth and health than is birth weight alone.

Important differences exist between babies that are born small for their gestational age and those that are of appropriate size. In general, babies born small for their gestational age have received fewer nutrients while in the uterus. Thus, they have a poorer mental and physical development record. Although it is not clear why, studies have also shown that small-for-gestational-age babies are more often hyperactive as children.

The likelihood of delivering a baby who is too small for his or her gestational age is much higher for teen-agers and for women of all ages who enter pregnancy underweight or undernourished, or who fail to gain enough weight during pregnancy.

We have come a long way in our understanding and appreciation of the role nutrition plays in the birth of healthy babies. It can now be said unequivocally that if you eat well before and during pregnancy and follow your weight gain carefully, you will be giving your child a healthy advantage at birth—an advantage that he or she will carry into childhood and beyond.

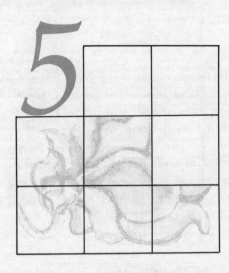

Gaining the Right Amount of Weight

Sue is five months pregnant now and waiting for her third appointment at the clinic. She doesn't mind the wait because it means that the inevitable will be delayed. She won't have to stand on the scales and be weighed quite yet. Last month the doctor said she was gaining too much weight and she had "better cut down." The thought of being scolded about her weight gain at this visit had sent Sue on a week-long, semi-starvation diet. It was a very tough week. Sue had a terrific appetite and was ready to eat anything. Now she is wondering how much her shoes and sweater weigh. She decided that this time she would take them off before she is weighed. Ten steps later and Sue is standing on the scale. The agony was worth it. She lost two pounds and won't be chided about her weight this time!

"How much weight should I gain?" It's a question every pregnant woman asks. Another—and better—way of asking the question is, "How much should my baby weigh at birth?" For that's the main reason to keep close tabs on your weight during pregnancy. You want to gain the amount of weight that offers the best assurance of producing a baby between seven pounds, fourteen ounces and nine pounds, the birth-weight range that promises the healthiest babies.

As noted in the previous chapter, three major factors will influence how much your baby weighs at birth. The first is the baby's gestational age. The longer your child remains in your womb, the more pounds he or she is likely to weigh at birth. Second is the amount of weight you gain during pregnancy. In general, the more weight you gain, the larger your baby will be. Third is your pre-pregnancy weight. If you begin your pregnancy underweight, you have a greater chance of delivering a smaller-than-average baby or a premature one. Overweight women, on the other hand, tend to have larger babies than normal-weight women even if they gain the same number of pounds. It seems their babies simply have more to grow on.

How Much Weight Gain is Right for Me?

There is no one weight-gain figure that's right for every woman. The amount of weight you should gain depends on how much you weighed before you became pregnant. Check the "Recommended Weight

Recommended Weight Goals during Pregnancy

Height without Shoes	Pre-Pregnancy Weight		
	Underweight If You Weighed This or Less	Normal Weight Range*	Overweight If You Weighed This or More
4'10"	88	89-108	109
4'11"	91	92-112	113
5'	94	95-115	116
5'1"	99	100-121	122
5'2"	104	105-127	128
5'3"	108	109-132	133
5'4"	113	114-138	139
5'5"	118	119-144	145
5'6"	123	124-150	151
5'7"	127	128-155	156
5'8"	132	133-161	162
5'9"	137	138-167	168
5'10"	142	143-173	174
5'11"	146	147-178	179
6'	151	152-184	185

*Normal weight for "thin-boned" women will be closer to the lower end of this range. For "big-boned" women, it will be closer to the higher end.

Your recommended weight gain goal for pregnancy:	Underweight 28-36 lbs.	Normal Weight 24-32 lbs.	Overweight 20-24 lbs.

Goals during Pregnancy" chart on page 40 to see if you were underweight, overweight, or at normal weight before your pregnancy.

A total weight gain of twenty-four to thirty-two pounds is recommended if you entered pregnancy at normal weight. If you entered it underweight you should, for the health of your baby and yourself, gain twenty-eight to thirty-six pounds. If you began your pregnancy overweight, you should gain twenty to twenty-four pounds.

Lower weight gains are all right for overweight women because a baby can get part of the calories he or she needs from the mother's existing "maternal energy stores" (a medical euphemism for "fat"). But—and this is very important—*you should not try to lose weight or seriously cut down on your eating while pregnant.* If you are a chronic dieter and perpetually overweight, this may be difficult to accept. It may even be difficult for your health-care provider to accept. But it is clear that your baby will be better off if you gain an appropriate amount of weight while eating nourishing foods.

At the other end of the scale is the problem of gaining too much weight. Unless you were very underweight before pregnancy or are carrying twins or triplets, gaining more than forty pounds will not make you or your baby healthier. It will just make it more difficult for you to lose the extra pounds later. If you *are* carrying more than one child, you should try to gain at least ten pounds more than the weight gain recommended on the weight-gain chart.

Where Does the Weight Gain Go?

The weight you gain during the first half of your pregnancy will be distributed throughout your body differently from that gained later. The first pounds will go into building up stores of fat and protein that can be used by your baby later in the pregnancy. Some of these stores will be held in reserve even longer to help meet your nutritional requirements after pregnancy and to help produce breastmilk. Nature assumes that humans, like other mammals, will breastfeed and wisely stores energy and nutrient supplies.

Other parts of your body will also be growing during the early months of your pregnancy. Your blood plasma will increase in quantity by almost fifty percent, as will other body fluids. Your breasts will begin to grow in anticipation of feeding the baby after birth and by midpregnancy will weigh about a pound more than before pregnancy.

And your uterus, of course, will become bigger. All of this growth puts on weight.

During the second half of your pregnancy, your stores of fat will decrease as the baby uses them for growth. But other parts of your body will be changing and making up that lost weight. Two membranes, known as the bag of waters or amniotic sac, will fill with about two pounds of amniotic fluid. This fluid helps cushion the fetus. The placenta, or afterbirth, which provides the fetus with food and oxygen, will also grow significantly during the last half of pregnancy. And, or course, the fetus itself will be getting bigger daily.

If you gain, say, twenty-nine pounds by the end of your pregnancy, those pounds will be distributed in approximately the following way:

	Weight in Pounds
Baby	8.5
Stores of fat and protein	7.5
Blood	4.0
Tissue fluids	2.7
Uterus (womb)	2.0
Amniotic fluid (bag of waters)	1.8
Placenta (afterbirth) and umbilical cord	1.5
Breasts	1.0
Total	29.0

Pacing the Weight Gain

If you are healthy and of normal weight at the start of your pregnancy, you can expect to gain at least ten pounds during the first twenty weeks and about a pound a week during the last twenty. Your appetite will probably be strongest between the tenth and thirtieth weeks of pregnancy. After that, your appetite will most likely taper off— and so will your rate of weight gain. You should, however, try to eat enough to maintain a gradual weight gain until you deliver your baby.

"My Weight Gain" charts to help you track your weight gain during pregnancy appear on pages 43-45. Select one of these charts, depending on whether you were overweight, underweight, or of normal weight before you became pregnant. (See "Recommended Weight Goals during Pregnancy" on page 40 to learn which group you are in.)

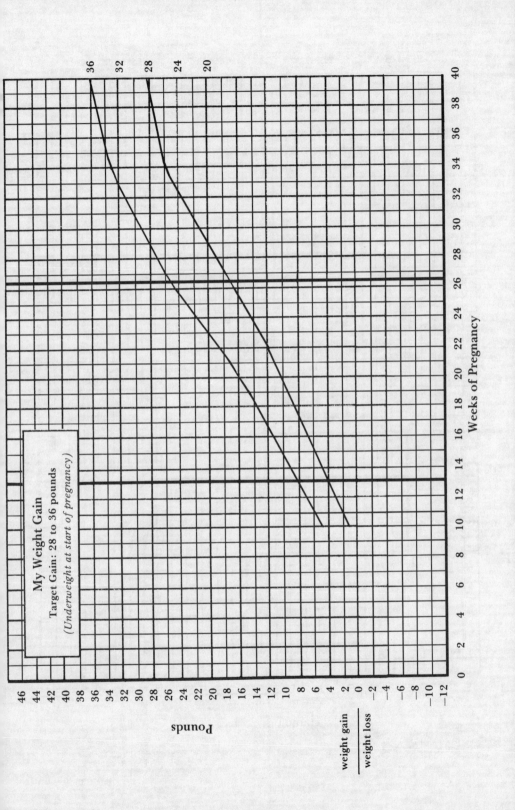

My Weight Gain
Target Gain: 28 to 36 pounds
(Underweight at start of pregnancy)

Pounds

46
44
42
40
38
36
34
32
30
28
26
24
22
20
18
16
14
12
10
8
6
4
2
0
−2
−4
−6
−8
−10
−12

weight gain
weight loss

0 2 4 6 8 10 12 14 16 18 20 22 24 26 28 30 32 34 36 38 40

Weeks of Pregnancy

36
32
28
24
20

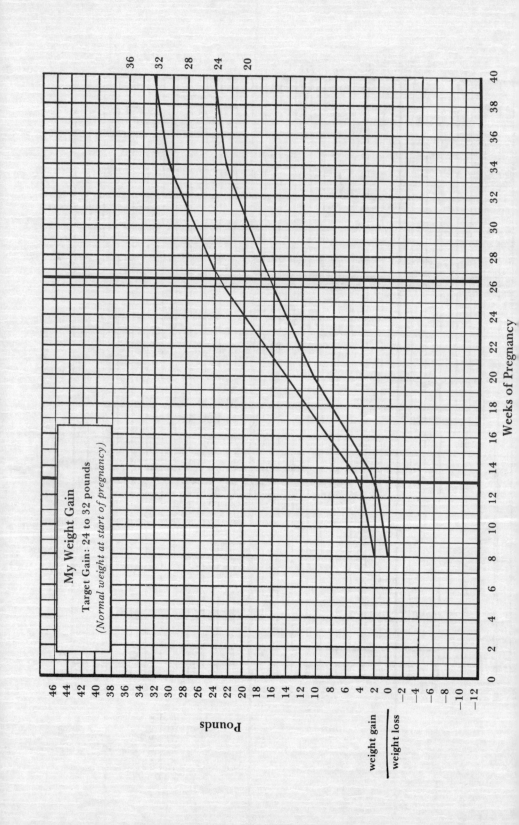

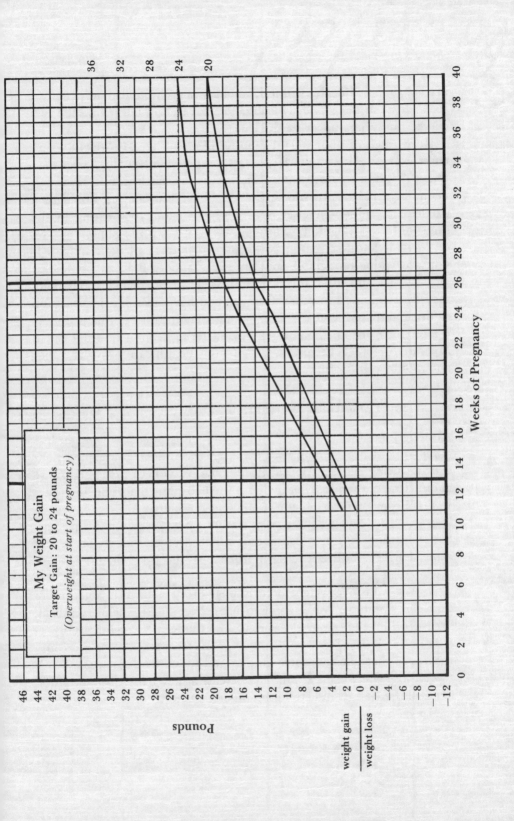

Mark a dot on the chart to indicate how many pounds you've gained so far in your pregnancy. Ideally, the dot should fall within the two curved lines that appear on the chart.

Keep track of your weight gain by filling in the "My Weight Gain" chart every week or two. If you discover you are gaining faster than the curve, don't launch into a diet! You can eat less, but be sure to maintain a balance of foods. Consider exercising more; walking is a particularly good exercise. *Never* cut down on your eating to the point of losing weight. Try, instead, to slow down the gain.

There is another reason to keep regular track of your weight. If you are eating moderately but are gaining more than two pounds a week, especially after the twentieth week of pregnancy, your body may be retaining too much fluid. If you have been cutting back on calories and find you are still gaining weight rapidly, this is double reason for caution, for you may be suffering from a disorder called *preeclampsia* (See Chapter 7). Tell your health-care provider about any rapid weight gain.

How Long Will It Take to Return to My Normal Weight?

Although maternity wards are by far the most successful weight-loss clinics in the world, you won't lose *all* the weight you gained right away. During the first week after delivery, you can expect to lose about fifteen pounds. That includes the baby, the placenta, and extra fluids. From then on, if you're nursing the baby, you can expect to lose at least a half pound a week rather effortlessly. On the average, breast-feeding mothers lose about twenty-five pounds by six weeks after delivery. Bottle-feeding mothers, on the other hand, tend to lose about twenty-one pounds.

If you were overweight before pregnancy, or if you gained more than forty pounds, you're going to be overweight after delivery. Again, breast-feeding can make it easier to lose that extra weight. If you decide not to breast-feed, make a conscious effort to exercise more and eat less so that you're losing half a pound to one pound a week. Don't try to lose the weight too quickly. With a new baby around, you'll need all the energy and strength you can muster.

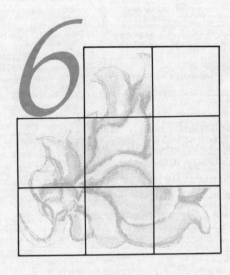

Getting You and
Your Life-Style
in Shape

*"Honey?" calls a voice from the kitchen. "Did you do your exercises today?"
Arlene pauses to think a moment. She isn't sure how to respond. All she knows
is that she's very tired and had planned to go to bed as soon as she finished fold-
ing the laundry. It's been a long day for her, and finding the energy to do her
exercises seems tough. But she isn't sure she wants the guilt associated with not
doing them either.*

*Arlene finally says what she's been thinking. "Joe, are you sure these exer-
cises help?"*

*"You know what our instructor said," replies Joe. "You'll be glad you stayed
in shape."*

*Giving a silent vow to keep her muscles in tone and have blood vessels down
to the tips of her toes, Arlene abandons the laundry and begins.*

Pregnancy is a great time to kick old, unhealthful habits and to culti-
vate new, healthful ones. It's a time, also, to slow down and take a
close look at how you live. What kind of unnecessary health risks do
you take in your life? Do you needlessly put yourself under stress?
Do you get enough rest and exercise?

Many of the things we do—or don't do—in our daily lives can harm
us, things like smoking and drinking, or failing to exercise or get

enough rest. Unfortunately, when these habits are continued during pregnancy, they harm not only the expectant mother but her unborn baby as well.

Every mother wants her baby to have the best possible start in life. So far, this book has talked primarily about how you can give your child a nutritional advantage at birth by improving your diet during pregnancy. Some of the topics discussed in this chapter also deal directly with food. But most deal with nutrition in its broad definition as "the act or process of nourishing or being nourished." Improving your habits is an important and loving way to "nourish" the baby you're carrying.

Smoking

One of your primary goals during pregnancy should be to deliver a baby that weighs somewhere between seven pounds, fourteen ounces and nine pounds, the range considered the most advantageous for a baby's future health and development (see Chapter 4). Smoking will hinder you in reaching this goal. This is especially true if, in addition to smoking, you follow a poor diet or fail to gain enough weight during your pregnancy.

Why? Because smoking lowers the amount of oxygen that reaches the fetus through the placenta. It may also reduce the amount of nutrients available to the fetus. As a result, babies born to women who smoke tend to be smaller than average. Fortunately, smoking does not appear to increase the risk of delivering a baby with malformations or other health problems unrelated to the birth weight of the infant.

If ever there was a time you should give up smoking, it is when you are pregnant. If you cannot quit, cut back on the number of cigarettes you smoke each day. Studies have shown that the more cigarettes a woman smokes during her pregnancy, the lower the birth weight of her child. Quitting smoking will also help your baby after he or she is born. Infants of smoking parents tend to come down with more respiratory illnesses than those of nonsmoking parents.

Alcohol

There is no absolutely safe amount of alcohol you can drink during pregnancy. Studies have shown that frequent consumption of two or more alcoholic drinks a day increases the risk of delivering a baby with physical and developmental abnormalities. For some women, even smaller amounts of alcohol may present the same risk. Occasional "binge" drinking, especially very early in pregnancy, also threatens the health of the fetus.

Alcohol should be avoided during pregnancy. For many pregnant women, abstention is a pleasure rather than a disappointment. They find pregnancy makes them lose their taste for alcoholic beverages, especially beer and wine. It is not clear why such taste changes occur, but they may be related to the increased production of the hormone *estrogen* during pregnancy.

Drugs

Many common drugs that are usually helpful and harmless can poison an unborn baby. Drugs have their most toxic effect on the fetus during the first half of pregnancy. During this period the fetus forms distinct organs and tissues (arms, heart, brain, kidneys, and legs) and is, therefore, most susceptible to outside factors—like drugs—that can cause malformations. After the fourth month, drugs have a greater chance of negatively affecting the fetus's general growth and development, rather than particular organs.

The sedative *thalidomide*, for example, which was prescribed to thousands of women, mostly European, in the 1950s and 1960s with tragic results, was most likely to produce malformations when it was taken between the twentieth and thirty-sixth days of pregnancy. Another sedative, *valium*, which continues to be taken by millions of women, has been linked to an increased risk of birth defects when used during the first three months of pregnancy. When taken during the last half of pregnancy, valium—as well as other sedatives—is associated with growth problems for the fetus.

Sedatives aren't the only drugs to be cautious about during pregnancy. The fact is *no drug—either over-the-counter or prescribed—has been proven absolutely safe to be taken during pregnancy*. Very little is known about how drugs affect fetal development. Tracing a birth defect to a specific cause is almost impossible. The effect of a particular drug on a fetus may depend on many factors, such as how much was taken and for how long.

To be safe, you should try to avoid medications during pregnancy.

This includes common over-the-counter drugs, such as laxatives, diuretics, cough medicines, and aspirin. Aspirin, for example, should be avoided especially during the last half of pregnancy because it can cause a delay in blood clotting. Aspirin substitutes do not appear to pose a similar threat.

Sometimes, the benefits of taking a drug outweigh the risks. Some drugs are necessary during pregnancy, either to relieve serious discomfort or to treat an illness. Let your health-care provider advise you. Never self-medicate during pregnancy.

Illicit drugs such as marijuana, cocaine, and LSD should also be avoided during pregnancy. Because the use of these drugs often goes hand-in-hand with other harmful habits, their effect on fetuses has been difficult to isolate. So far, however, these drugs do not appear to have a more dramatic harmful effect on fetuses than legally prescribed drugs. All should be avoided.

Caffeine

Most of the caffeine we consume comes from coffee, cocoa, tea, and cola beverages. Caffeine can also be found in pain relievers and over-the-counter diet pills. The side-effects of too much caffeine—nervousness, difficulty in sleeping, and a frequent need to urinate—are well known to those who drink large amounts of coffee. These are also some of the side-effects of pregnancy. So when you put caffeine and pregnancy together, you increase these problems.

Moderate amounts of caffeine (fewer than four cups of coffee or four cola beverages a day) do not seem to threaten fetuses. However, some studies with animals have indicated that larger amounts of caffeine may produce birth defects. The final verdict is not yet in; to be on the safe side try to reduce your consumption of caffeine to less than 500 milligrams a day. Better yet, give it up. Caffeine beverages don't really contribute anything good to your diet except water, and you can get that from healthier sources, such as vegetable juices, fruit juices, or water.

Below is a list of foods and their caffeine content.

Food	Caffeine Content
Brewed coffee (3/4)	125 mg.
Strong tea (3/4) cup)	89 mg.
Instant iced-tea (3/4 cup)	72 mg.
Instant coffee (3/4 cup)	64 mg.

Cocoa (3/4 cup)	60 mg.
Instant tea (3/4 cup)	55 mg.
Cola (12 oz.)	52 mg.
Weak tea (3/4 cup)	33 mg.
Decaffeinated coffee (3/4 cup)	3 mg.
Milk chocolate candy (1 oz.)	3 mg.

Saccharin

Saccharin is an artificial sweetener used in many "diet" food products, especially diet soft drinks. Whether it should be prohibited during pregnancy is still being debated by scientists. The available evidence, however, suggests that the frequent use of products containing saccharin may cause cancer. Until more studies are done, you should avoid this sweetener during pregnancy. Besides, products that contain saccharin usually fail to contribute anything worthwhile to your diet.

Hazards Outside the Home

It is estimated that more than half of the women who become pregnant in America work at least up through their seventh month of pregnancy. There is no reason for them not to work—as long as they and the conditions they are working under are healthy.

Many pregnant working women, unfortunately, come into daily contact with toxic substances that can present serious health risks to their fetus, especially during the first half of pregnancy when the fetus is developing its internal organs. These potentially hazardous substances include herbicides, pesticides, solvents (especially benzene), and toxic gases, fumes, and vapors. You should avoid exposure to these during pregnancy. You should also try to avoid x-rays. If you must have an x-ray, make sure your abdomen is protected with a lead shield. High doses of radiation can result in birth defects. Long-term exposure to low doses of radiation may also cause birth defects. If your job brings you into close contact with radiation or radioactive materials, be sure you are thoroughly protected.

Hazards Inside the Home

Many of the products you use routinely in your home should be avoided or used with extreme caution during pregnancy. These include garden insecticides and herbicides, turpentine, furniture stripper, and aerosol spray products that are propelled by fluorocarbons. The fumes from these products can be absorbed into your body through your skin or lungs and then passed on to your unborn child. Paint fumes are also dangerous; so avoid painting during pregnancy, especially if you are using an oil-based paint.

Pregnant women should also avoid changing cat litters. Cats can be carriers of an infection called toxoplasmosis, which, if developed by a pregnant woman, can result in a miscarriage, a stillbirth, or birth defects.

A number of potentially hazardous substances also enter our homes on or in the foods we eat. Of particular concern for pregnant women are foods contaminated with herbicides, pesticides, mercury, and lead.

A great debate exists concerning foods grown with herbicides and pesticides and whether they pose a health threat to those who eat them. Many people prefer to play it safe by eating only organically grown food (food that has been cultivated without the use of chemicals). Unfortunately, this food is often expensive or difficult to find. Another solution is to carefully wash all the fruits and vegetables you bring into your home in a mild detergent solution. This way you will be removing any external residue of herbicides or pesticides.

Two major environmental contaminants, PCB's (polychlorinated biphenyls) and PBB's (polybrominated biphenyls) pose a clearer risk to pregnant women. Studies have shown that babies born to pregnant women who have been exposed to PCB's or PBB's have a higher-than-average incidence of physical abnormalities.

PCB's and PBB's are used in the manufacture of plastics and flame retardants. During pregnancy you should avoid any job that brings you in direct contact with these chemicals. Unfortunately, through improper use of storage, PCB's and PBB's sometimes turn up where they are not supposed to and, as a result, contaminate foods that enter our homes. In 1973, for example, Michigan cows were accidentally fed PBB. Before the mistake was uncovered, millions of Michigan residents had drunk contaminated milk.

Although they are rare, such outbreaks of PCB and PBB contamination do occur. Most often it is a water supply that is polluted. People are exposed to the chemicals by eating fish they caught in the contaminated water. Before you go fishing, check with your State Health Department for information about sites in your state that are contaminated.

Mercury and lead, when ingested through food, also pose a health threat to an unborn child. Mercury poisoning can cause blindness and mental retardation; lead poisoning can instigate a spontaneous abortion. Like PCB's and PBB's, mercury poisoning usually occurs as a result of eating fish caught in contaminated water. Often warnings are posted not to fish in such waters, but you should double-check with your State Health Department.

Fortunately, lead exposure seems to be on the decline, largely because of new regulations that control lead in such products as gasoline. Lead poisoning still sometimes occurs, however, when unglazed pots and dishes coated with a lead-based paint are used in the preparation and serving of food.

Exercise

Maintaining the same level of physical fitness during pregnancy that you were used to before pregnancy can become a challenge. But there are advantages to staying physically fit. Chances are that you will feel better during pregnancy, have a better emotional outlook and attitude, resist disease better, sleep better, and eat better if you exercise regularly. Your labor may be shorter and less stressful. You will likely recover more quickly from labor and delivery than if you decided to cash in your membership at the YWCA.

You should keep in mind several precautions when considering the amount and type of exercise appropriate for you. These precautions are intended not to make you fearful of exercising during pregnancy, but to help you make sensible decisions about which exercises to pursue.

If you were out-of-shape before you became pregnant, don't suddenly go on a "crash program" of strenuous exercising. You need to exercise, but begin moderately to avoid putting undue stress on you and your baby.

If you were following an exercise program before you became pregnant, you can probably continue with that program. Just leave out activities that make you susceptible to jolting or falling, such as horseback riding, sky-diving, and down-hill skiing. Although your baby is well-protected by a resilient uterus and a cushion of amniotic fluid, he or she is vulnerable to the impact of a major fall.

Falling comes easier to pregnant women, especially during exercises and activities that require a keen sense of balance. The problem, of course, is that as your stomach "grows" your center of balance changes. Toward the end of a pregnancy, this can create some difficult balancing acts. Have you ever watched a woman in her ninth month of pregnancy struggle to get up from a deep, soft chair? Or try to regain her balance after losing her footing on a slippery sidewalk? The change in your center of gravity takes some getting used to.

Don't overdo your exercising. Several studies have indicated that very high levels of physical work and exercise may reduce infant birth weight and vitality. With so much energy and nutrients going to meet the needs of the mother's activities, not enough may be left for the rapidly developing baby. When you over-exercise you may also end up with two temporary chemical waste products (lactic acid and ketone bodies) in your body that may be harmful to the baby.

Most pregnant women, however, should worry more about under-exercising than over-exercising. So don't look for excuses. Go forth and exercise sensibly. Substitute walking for riding in a car or bus. Continue to jog if you're used to it. Take time each day to do some bending and stretching exercises. And put into your schedule swimming, volleyball, tennis, or other sports that you enjoy.

The basic type of exercise you can pursue during pregnancy is aerobic exercise, which requires a steady stream of oxygen over a sustained period of time. Aerobic exercise helps your heart and lungs work more efficiently, which contributes to your endurance and overall health. Following is a list of aerobic activities. To get the most out of these activities, you should engage in them three to five times a week.

> Walking
> Swimming
> Bicycling
> Tennis
> Volleyball
> Badminton
> Jogging
> Cross-country skiing

Walking and swimming are by far the best exercises to do when you are pregnant—especially if you began your pregnancy out-of-shape. More vigorous aerobic activities, such as cross-country skiing and jogging, should be pursued during pregnancy only by women who are used to them or who are already reasonably physically fit.

The other type of exercise you should do regularly involves bending and stretching. Several examples of these exercises are illustrated on pages 56 and 57. Bending and stretching exercises will help get you in shape for labor and delivery by increasing your flexibility, muscular strength, and endurance. They will also help you relax and sleep better. You should do these exercises daily.

You'll probably notice that physical activity tends to be more tiring during your pregnancy than it was before pregnancy. One reason for the increased tiredness is the additional weight you are carrying. Another reason is the increased amount of blood pumping through your body. Tiring easily is usually most noticeable around the third month of pregnancy when your blood volume increases substantially and around the last month when your weight is at its greatest.

Don't let this discourage you from exercising. In the long run, exercising sensibly and regularly will give you more energy during pregnancy, not less.

Stress

Women who experience serious psychological stress during pregnancy tend to deliver babies with lower birth weights than those who are not under stress. Their babies also tend to have more health problems. Also, stress can create a greater susceptibility to disease for the mother.

For the health of your baby as well as yourself, you should attempt to eliminate as many stressful factors during pregnancy as you can. Learn how to pace your life so you are not rushing from one project or activity to another. Take time to relax and rest. During pregnancy you should be getting at least eight hours of sleep each night. You may want to take additional rests when you feel you need them, especially during the second and third months of pregnancy when your energy level is usually lowest.

One way to resist the harmful effects of stress is by eating well. Stress leads to a quicker breakdown of protein, carbohydrates, and fats within the body; it also increases the need for vitamin C. A well-balanced diet rich in vitamin C can replenish these lost nutrients and help keep the stress you are experiencing from leading to illness. Being physically fit can also help you resist the effects of stress.

Exercises during Pregnancy

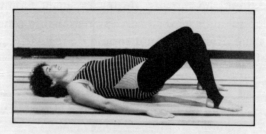

Pelvic tilt: Lie on floor with knees bent. Tighten buttock and stomach muscles. Push your back flat against the floor. Hold for three seconds, then relax.

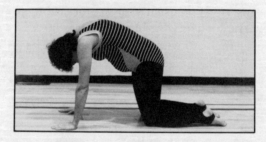

Cat stretch: Get on your hands and knees with back straight. Pull up your pelvis and arch your back like a cat. Hold for a few seconds, then relax into a straight-back position.

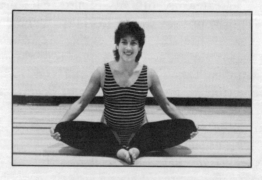

Hip stretch: Sit with soles of feet pressed together. Place a hand under each knee. Using your thigh muscles, press your knees down toward the floor. At the same time, try to pull up on your knees with your hands. Keep up the resistance for a few seconds, then relax.

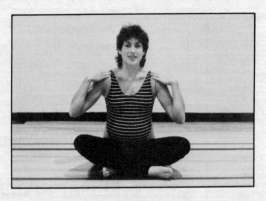

Shoulder rolls: Sit on the floor with your knees bent and your ankles crossed. Place your hands on your shoulders. Rotate your shoulders in circles, first forward, then backward. Relax.

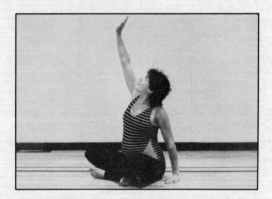

Arm stretch: Sit on the floor with your knees bent and ankles crossed. Stretch one arm, then the other above your head. Reach as high as you can, then relax.

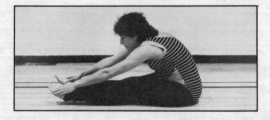

Leg stretch: Sit on floor with legs slightly apart. Stretch forward slowly and attempt to touch your toes. Hold this forward position, then slowly sit back up and relax.

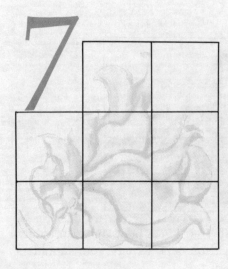

7

Dietary Aids for Common Problems

"There are some very unromantic aspects to this pregnancy business," re-marked Pam to her friend Carol. "I'm thrilled at the thought of having a baby. We're really looking forward to it," Pam said. "But, it hasn't gone exactly the way I expected."

"How's that?" asked Carol.

"Well," said Pam, "nobody ever told me that pregnant women get heartburn, constipation, and food cravings. Or that morning sickness can last all day. I ex-pected mine to be a normal pregnancy. Now I know that these problems are nor-mal during pregnancy for lots of women."

"Okay, then," said Carol. "Why are you so upset?"

"Because," answered Pam, "nobody told me about them until after *they happened."*

Many women experience bothersome problems that are part of a normal pregnancy. Most problems are easily managed with proper self-care or medical attention. Few women are spared the experience of one problem or another that they did not expect.

Diet can help keep many of the common problems of pregnancy under control, as you'll discover while reading this chapter. However, before you follow any of the suggestions made here, discuss them with your health-care provider.

Morning Sickness

Morning sickness, or nausea, can occur at any time during the day, but it is most often experienced right after waking up in the morning. Almost half of all pregnant women experience nausea during the first three months of pregnancy. Fortunately, the problem usually disappears after that. If it continues beyond the third month, and especially if it is accompanied by vomiting, you should get medical attention.

Here are some dietary ways you can help ease the symptoms of nausea:

- Keep a stack of dry crackers next to your bed and eat a few before you get out of bed in the morning. (You may also want to keep a wisk broom handy to clear the cracker crumbs off your sheets.)
- Start the day in slow motion. Get out of bed slowly and avoid sudden movements.
- Drink liquids between meals, rather than with meals.
- Eat small, frequent meals. Nausea becomes more intense when the stomach is empty.
- Avoid foods and odors that bring on the feeling of nausea. Fried foods, coffee, beer, and strongly flavored vegetables are frequent culprits.
- Turn instead to starchy foods, such as bread, pastas, potatoes, and crackers, which are usually well tolerated during bouts of nausea.
- Consume foods that are good sources of vitamin B_6. (See on page 99 in the appendix for good sources of this vitamin.)

A supplement of vitamin B_6 is often prescribed as a treatment for nausea. If you take a B_6 supplement, you should experience less nausea within two weeks. If the nausea doesn't improve by then, the vitamin B_6 supplement will probably not help you. Why vitamin B_6 relieves nausea for some women and not for others remains a mystery. Perhaps it helps some women by replenishing a B_6 deficiency. However, because of the size of the dose usually prescribed—about nineteen times the normal RDA levels—it's more likely that the B_6 acts as a medication rather than as a vitamin.

Women with morning sickness frequently have a weight-gain problem. Some gain weight too fast as a result of overeating; they have found that lessens their nausea. Others lose weight because the nausea makes food seem repugnant or because it leads to vomiting. If you are experiencing nausea, carefully plan your diet around foods and beverages that won't aggravate the condition. Remember, it's important for the future health of your baby that you gain weight at a steady, gradual pace.

Constipation

Constipation is a frequent complaint of many Americans, but it is even more common during pregnancy when the hormone *progesterone* is released into the body in high amounts. Progesterone causes the muscles of the intestines to lose some of their strength. As a result, passage of food through the intestines slows down. Toward the end of pregnancy, the weight of the fetus pressing down on the intestines may also contribute to constipation. Other factors that can aggravate the condition are a low-fiber diet, inadequate exercise, and a low consumption of liquids.

If constipation is not relieved—especially during the last few months of pregnancy—painful hemorrhoids may occur.

You can help keep constipation under control by eating foods rich in fiber. The value of fiber lies in its ability to absorb water. By attracting water, fiber makes stools bulkier and softer, enabling them to move more easily through the intestines. (If you have ever let a bowl of bran cereal and milk sit on a table for a few minutes, you know how quickly fiber attracts fluids.)

The average American consumes about six grams of fiber each day. This is much lower than the twelve to fifteen grams recommended to prevent constipation. Following is a list of foods and their comparative fiber content.

Food	Serving Size	Amount of Fiber (Grams)
Bran cereals (not flakes)	1/2 cup	10 to 13
Parsnips, cooked	1/2 cup	5.5
Green peas, cooked	1/2 cup	5.5
Rolled oats, dry	1/2 cup	5.0
Grits, dry	1/4 cup	5.0
Cracked wheat, dry	1/3 cup	5.0
Dried beans, cooked	1/2 cup	4.5
Carrots, cooked	1/2 cup	3.7
Shredded wheat	1 large biscuit	3.0
Whole wheat bread	1 slice	2.7
Cabbage, cooked	1/2 cup	2.7

Pear	1 small	2.4
Strawberries	1/2 cup	2.1
Banana	1 medium	1.8
Plum, raw	2	1.5
Apple	1 small	1.4
White bread	1 slice	0.8

It is possible to include too much fiber in your diet. Excess amounts (more than about fifteen grams per day) can lead to diarrhea and the incomplete absorption of nutrients from food. Of particular concern is the loss of fluid and of the minerals zinc, iron, calcium, and magnesium. But for most people eating too much fiber is not as much a problem as eating too little.

Besides eating high-fiber foods, constipation can be eased by drinking plenty of fluids—at least ten servings a day—and exercising regularly. If the problem becomes severe, laxatives can help. However, you should take laxatives only under the supervision of your health-care provider. Certain types of laxatives can cause diarrhea, which in turn may cause you to lose an excessive amount of minerals.

Heartburn

Heartburn is a common problem that usually pops up toward the end of pregnancy. It results primarily from the baby pressing on the stomach. Such pressure can cause food and digestive juices in the stomach to spurt up into the esophagus. It's called heartburn because you feel the pain near your heart.

To avoid heartburn, try to keep your stomach from getting full. Small, frequent meals will usually do the trick.

Antacids that you might not hesitate to use for indigestion before pregnancy should be taken with caution during pregnancy. Some antacids contain undesirably large amounts of minerals.

Leg Cramps

A leg cramp can be a rude awakening for a pregnant woman. Such cramps occur most frequently at night and usually involve the calf muscles of the leg.

Scientists aren't sure what causes leg cramps during pregnancy. One theory suggests that cramps may result from a calcium or sodium deficiency in the body. But that theory remains unproven.

You may be able to decrease the incidence of leg cramps by eating a well-balanced diet and by drinking plenty of fluids. When a cramp does occur, increase blood circulation at the site of the cramp by massaging the muscle or applying a warm compress. Vitamin and mineral supplements have *not* been shown to be helpful in preventing leg cramps.

Poor Appetite

A poor appetite can become a problem if it leads to an unbalanced diet, a weight loss during the first three months of pregnancy, or a failure to gain weight at an appropriate rate after that.

Poor appetite has many causes. A vitamin and mineral deficiency can powerfully reduce your desire for food. So, of course, can nausea and vomiting.

If you are suffering from a poor appetite you should examine your diet carefully. Check to make sure you are eating foods rich in all the vitamins and minerals you need. (See "My Daily Vitamin and Mineral Needs" chart on pages 15-17.) Eating small, frequent meals can also be a way of matching your food needs with your weak appetite.

Sometimes a prenatal vitamin and mineral supplement or a B-complex vitamin supplement can help improve a poor appetite. Talk to your health-care provider about it.

Excessive Appetite

Eating too much food can also occur during pregnancy. If you find that you are consistently overweight during your pregnancy by five or more pounds (see "Target Weight Gain" charts on pages 43-45), you should try to curb your appetite.

Your goal, however, should be to slow down the rate of your weight gain. As stated before, you should never try to lose weight during pregnancy.

The best way to slow down your weight gain is by eating less and exercising more. Review the "My Diet" chart you filled out in Chapter 1. Decide which low-nutrient, high-calorie foods you can eliminate from your diet and which you can eat in smaller amounts. Then sit down and plan a new healthful diet—and stick to the plan. Planned diets are better than making spontaneous food choices—especially if your food choices are usually made when you're hungry or in a hurry.

You can also help slow down an excessive gain of weight during pregnancy by exercising more. Below is a list of activities and the number of calories each burns off in an hour. The figures assume that you weigh 150 pounds. If you weigh less, you will burn off fewer calories during an hour; if you weigh more, you will burn off additional calories.

Activity	Calories Burned per Hour
Sitting	100
Standing	140
Housework	180
Walking slowly (2½ mph)	210
Bicycling slowly (5½ mph)	210
Gardening	220
Golfing	250
Mowing lawn	250
Walking medium fast (3 to 4 mph)	300
Swimming	300
Square dancing	350
Volleyball	350
Tennis	420
Bicycling fast (13 mph)	630
Running (10 mph)	900

Remember, exercise and eating less go hand in hand. To reduce your rate of weight gain by a pound a week, you must decrease the calories you take in *and* increase the calories you expend to 3500 calories per week. For example, you could eat 1400 fewer calories per week and burn off 2100 calories by swimming an hour a day. Total: 3500 calories. The combinations are endless. But don't overdo it to the point where you're actually losing weight.

Food Cravings

Many pregnant women experience food cravings. Contrary to popular opinion, these cravings are not related to emotional insecurity or the need for attention. Research has shown that eighty-seven percent of normal, healthy, pregnant women report cravings for a variety of foods, including pizza, milk, cottage cheese, and, yes, even pickles. Some women develop a "sweet tooth" during pregnancy; others desire salty foods. Many women also report that foods they enjoyed before pregnancy — especially coffee, beer, and beef — are now repugnant to smell or taste.

Why food cravings develop and food preferences change during pregnancy is not clear. But they do happen — often before a woman even knows she is pregnant.

You shouldn't worry about food cravings, as long as they don't interfere with retaining a healthful, well-balanced diet. Some women, however, develop strong desires to eat non-food items, such as clay or laundry starch. These kinds of cravings have been reported since Biblical times. Needless to say, they can lead to serious health problems and should be strongly resisted.

Swelling

Almost eighty percent of pregnant women experience swelling, or edema, during their pregnancies. The swelling usually takes the form of "puffy ankles." Ankle swelling is caused by the fetus putting pressure on the blood vessels that lead to the mother's legs. This, in turn, causes fluid to move from the blood into the surrounding tissues. Eventually, the fluid gravitates to the lowest part of the body — the ankles.

Ankle swelling has *not* been linked to health problems. Only a few years ago, this type of swelling was aggressively treated by putting the pregnant woman on a low-calorie, salt-restricting diet, and by prescribing diuretics. However, these practices were found to be ineffective and even harmful, for they contributed to such real health threats as high blood pressure and low weight gain. They are no longer recommended.

Swelling is a cause for concern during pregnancy when it occurs in the hands or face. A fluid build-up in these parts of the body may indicate a blood circulation problem. You should inform your health-care provider if you notice that your hands or face are swelling.

The extra fluid you retain from swelling may show up as extra pounds on the scale, but that's no reason to go on a crash diet. Water weight is not caused by too many calories, so cutting back on a good diet will not reduce the swelling. In fact, it will probably make it worse.

To keep swelling under control, make sure you are not restricting your salt intake. Also, be sure to get enough protein—about seventy-four to 100 grams per day. Protein acts as a diuretic. It draws fluid into the blood, enabling the fluid to be excreted eventually by the kidney. Below is a list of foods and their protein content:

Food	Serving Size	Grams
Cottage Cheese (lowfat)	1 cup	28
Chicken (no skin)	3 oz.	27
Beef roast (lean)	3 oz.	25
Pork chop (lean)	3 oz.	25
Tuna	3 oz.	24
Beefsteak (lean)	3 oz.	24
Veal cutlet	3 oz.	23
Lamb (leg roast)	3 oz.	22
Liver (beef)	3 oz.	22
Shrimp	3 oz.	21
Hamburger	3 oz.	21
Fish (haddock)	3 oz.	19
Chili (with meat and beans)	1 cup	19
Ham	3 oz.	18
Sausage (pork links)	3 oz.	17
Beans (dried)	1 cup	15
Stew (beef and vegetable)	1 cup	15
Custard (baked)	1 cup	13
Lima beans	1 cup	12
Milk	1 cup	9
Peanuts	1/4 cup	9
Peanut butter	2 tablespoons	8
Eggs	1	6

Preeclampsia

When swelling of the ankles, hands, and feet is accompanied by high blood pressure and a spillage of protein into the urine, a disorder called preeclampsia is usually present. Preeclampsia primarily affects the kidney and circulatory system and is unique to pregnancy. It occurs in about seven percent of first pregnancies, and even less often in subsequent ones. The symptoms usually show themselves about half-way through a pregnancy. In serious cases, convulsions can occur. When this happens, the disorder is called eclampsia.

The cause of preeclampsia is unknown. But women who enter

pregnancy underweight, obese, or malnourished are more likely to develop it than well-nourished women of normal weight.

The swelling that accompanies preeclampsia can result in a rapid gain of weight—as much as seven "water" pounds by the time the swelling becomes obvious. In the past, such rapid weight gains were confused with overeating. As a result, pregnant women suffering from preeclampsia were often put on a low-calorie, salt-restricted diet and prescribed diuretics. This treatment did harm rather than good, for it reduced the growth of the fetus and did nothing for the preeclampsia. It is no longer recommended.

If you should develop preeclampsia, maintaining a well-balanced diet will help you keep it under control. Pay special attention to your protein intake. If necessary, it should be brought up to 100 grams per day. (See list of high-protein foods under "Swelling" section on page 65.)

Although high blood pressure is a symptom of preeclampsia and doctors recommend a salt-restricted diet for most non-pregnant patients suffering from high blood pressure, you should *not* restrict your salt intake when you develop preeclampsia. On the contrary, you should make sure you get enough salt by salting your foods to taste. High blood pressure that surfaces during pregnancy is not related to salt intake, but rather to hormonal changes. If, however, you *enter* pregnancy with high blood pressure, your health-care provider will probably—and properly—prescribe a salt-restricted diet and diuretics to keep it under control.

If you are suffering from preeclampsia, your health-care provider may prescribe plenty of bed rest. If the condition is serious, you may also have to deliver your baby by caesarean section to avoid problems associated with high blood pressure during labor and delivery, such as convulsions and coma.

Nutritional Anemias

Nutritional anemias occur when there is a shortage of one or more of the nutrients in the blood that are required to build red blood cells. During pregnancy, these anemias are usually the result of a poor overall diet or a deficiency of iron or folacin. A woman with anemia looks pale, tires easily, eats poorly, and is more likely to develop infections. Her baby has a greater chance of becoming anemic during his or her first year of life. Anemia occurs less often during a first pregnancy than in later ones when the body's nutrient stores may be near empty.

As part of your prenatal care, your health-care provider will check your blood periodically for signs of anemia. Either a hemoglobin or a hemotacrit analysis will be performed. A hemoglobin reading of less than eleven percent or a hematocrit reading of less than thirty-three percent indicates that anemia may exist.

The management of anemia caused by an iron or folacin deficiency calls for a well-balanced diet that contains foods rich in iron and folacin. Check the "Food Sources of Key Nutrients" chart on page 93 of the appendix for a list of the best food sources of these two nutrients. Try to eat at least two iron-rich and two folacin-rich foods each day. Consuming a well-balanced diet will also help prevent anemia from developing again.

In addition to eating a well-balanced diet, you should take iron and folacin supplements to help prevent anemia. One daily milligram of folacin is recommended; thirty to sixty milligrams of iron. If taken in large doses, iron can cause digestive problems, so it would be best to meet your daily iron requirement with three pills containing ten to twenty milligrams each rather than the entire daily dose. Each tablet should be taken between meals with a glass of orange juice. The vitamin C in the orange juice makes the iron easier to absorb. Iron tablets come in many forms, such as ferrous sulfate, ferrous gluconate, and ferrous fumarate. If you find that one type causes heartburn, gas, diarrhea, or contstipation, try another. Also, be sure to store your iron pills out of the reach of children; swallowing large amounts can be very dangerous.

There are many other types of anemia that may develop during pregnancy, all of them rare. Anemia resulting from a vitamin B_6 or B_{12} deficiency, a loss of blood, or an inherited condition can become a problem for a small percentage of pregnant women.

Diabetes

Diabetes occurs when the pancreas fails to produce enough of the hormone *insulin*. The body needs insulin to process its main fuel, the sugar *glucose*. Out of every 200 women who become pregnant, one is a diabetic. And four others will develop diabetes sometime during their pregnancy. This form of the disease is called *gestational diabetes*. Women who enter pregnancy obese or who have family members with diabetes are more likely to develop gestational diabetes during pregnancy.

Although it's not known why, women who have diabetes tend to deliver babies that weigh more than average at birth. Their babies also tend to be in poorer health at birth. Because of these factors, many doctors prefer to deliver the babies of diabetic women by caesarean section before they have reached full term. If you have diabetes, you should gain the same amount of weight during pregnancy as non-diabetic women. Good control of your blood-sugar levels will be the most important factor in the delivery of a healthy, normal-weight baby. It's extremely important, therefore, that you be under careful medical supervision throughout your pregnancy.

The management of diabetes involves balancing insulin shots (if taken), food intake, weight gain, physical activity, and blood-sugar levels. As a pregnant woman with diabetes, you need the same amounts of nutrients as other pregnant women. Actually, most diabetics take great care with their diets and have eating habits to be envied by their non-diabetic friends.

If you developed diabetes during pregnancy, you have a twenty to thirty percent chance of becoming diabetic again later in life. To reduce your risk of a diabetes recurrence, maintain normal weight, eat a balanced diet, and exercise regularly.

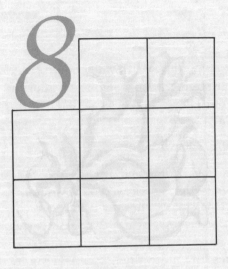

Nourishing Your Newborn and Yourself

At 6 a.m. the two-month-old Max-alarm goes off, right on schedule. Beth sleepily opens her eyes. Already she can feel her breastmilk "let down" in anticipation of the morning feeding. She tilts her head toward her husband, Bruce, who has also been wakened by the crying baby.

"I'll get him," Bruce says. A few seconds later he returns with Max. Beth takes the baby into her arms and offers him her breast which he takes eagerly.

Bruce begins to get ready for work. Half an hour later, he returns and asks Beth if she's ready for breakfast. Beth nods. Max is almost finished feeding.

Within a few minutes Beth can hear eggs sizzling in the kitchen. Noticing that Max has begun his morning nap, Beth asks herself "would I rather sleep or eat breakfast?" She doesn't have a chance to answer. Sleep comes before she can decide.

In many ways, being a new parent is an indescribable experience, bordering on the magical. Parts of the experience, however, can be described by such prosaic words as *busy, exhausting*, and *demanding*. In the days and weeks right after delivery, you'll find that many demands will be placed on your time and physical endurance. Things like eating a balanced diet may not be easy. But you shouldn't forsake a healthful diet after your child is born. This is also a time when you need to be nourishing your baby, either directly through breast-feeding or indirectly by regaining your strength and stamina. To nourish your baby, you need to nourish yourself.

Nourishing Yourself

After delivery, you may devote so much time and attention to your new baby and the rest of your family that you leave your own nourishing to chance. Many women, particularly those who breast-feed, forgo meals for the chance to get some rest. By not eating properly, a vicious cycle develops. You tire more easily, which leads you to eat even more erratically, which makes you more tired, etc. As a result, you are likely to become ill and need even more rest. Taking care to eat a well-balanced diet will help you avoid this downward cycle. It will also help you regain your stamina by replenishing the stores of nutrients that were depleted by pregnancy.

Keep Meals Simple

In the days following delivery, plan simple meals, such as sandwiches and soups, that can be prepared quickly. Keep on hand a stock of fresh fruits, canned fruits, crackers, juices, peanut butter, milk, and cheese for easy, nutritious snacking. Your partner's cooperation in the kitchen may also prove to be very helpful. The arrival of a new baby has given a lot of men the opportunity to blossom as cooks.

Vitamin and mineral supplements are probably not needed after the baby is born if you remained healthy during pregnancy. A well-balanced diet will provide all the nutrients you need. As a precaution, however, your health-care provider may advise you to take the same supplements you used during pregnancy for two or three months after delivery.

Nourishing Your Baby

All newborns, whether breastfed or bottlefed, have the same need for nutrients—a need that is greater now than it will ever be again. Yet fulfilling this need requires a very simple diet. Until at least the fourth month of life, a baby can be completely nourished by breastmilk or infant formula. Served with love and attention, this diet makes babies thrive.

A baby's great need for nutrients is a result of his or her rapid growth and development. For the first two months of life, a baby will gain about one ounce a day, or about a pound every two weeks. If growth proceeds on course, a baby's birth rate will triple and his or her length will increase by fifty percent by the end of the first year of life. This is an enormous rate of growth. If that pace were to continue beyond the first year, a five-year-old child would weigh more than seven tons and stand more than thirteen feet tall!

How much a baby will want to eat depends on his or her pattern of growth. Baby growth occurs in spurts, rather than at a gradual, constant pace. Babies will be noticeably more hungry right before a growth spurt. One very common pre-growth period occurs for most babies when they are fourteen to twenty-eight days old. So don't be shocked if your baby seems to want to eat all the time during those two weeks.

Because a baby naturally adjusts his or her appetite to the level needed for growth, you should feed your newborn whenever he or she is hungry. Feeding babies on a by-the-clock schedule may lead to undereating or overeating. Wait until your baby is six to nine months old before you attempt to fit his or her feedings into your family's meal schedule. By then, most babies can adjust to eating meals and snacks with the rest of the family. But always remain flexible; don't regiment your baby's eating times.

Because babies have a great need for nutrients and small stomachs, they get hungry often. During the first few weeks, your baby will probably want to eat every two or three hours. At each feeding, he or she will drink about two or three ounces of breastmilk or formula. By your baby's second month, the interval between his or her demands to be fed may stretch to three or four hours. By six months, most babies need to eat only five or six times per day.

Feedings should be followed by burpings. Babies swallow air along with their breastmilk or formula. After a meal, they receive considerable relief and comfort from a few gentle pats on the back.

Recognizing a Hungry Baby

Because babies cry for a variety of reasons, recognizing when a cry means hunger can be difficult. It is important, however, that you learn to identify the hunger cry. Babies will often eat when they are hungry because food, or the process of eating, is an acceptable substitute for what they really want. Eating for the wrong reason, however, can establish a poor pattern for later life.

Hungry babies feed with enthusiasm. They will shut out the rest of the world while they are eating. Hungry babies suck eagerly and quickly forget their discomfort as soon as they start to eat. A baby who really wants something other than food will suck on the bottle or breast half-heartedly and will be easily distracted.

Learning how to recognize a true "hunger cry" can take months — or years. Most children cannot identify or explain their hunger until they are about three years old. You will have to decide for your child when it is time to eat. So it's important to get the signals straight.

It is also important to recognize when a baby has had enough to eat. Many parents seem to suffer from "the more the baby eats the better we feel" syndrome. All too much time goes into coaxing a baby to finish that last ounce or two in a bottle, or to swallow that last bite of food. Learn to accept when your baby is no longer hungry. Don't force food on him or her. Remember, babies will eat when they're hungry and they'll stop eating when they're full.

If you are concerned that your baby may not be getting enough food, have your health-care provider check your baby's growth progress. If your baby is not growing at the rate expected, your health-care provider can then identify the reason why. A baby who does not get enough food and, as a result, grows at a slower-than-normal rate can experience permanent set-backs in growth and development.

Breast-Feeding

Breastmilk offers babies many more benefits than formula. It contains substances that provide protection from infectious diseases and allergies. It is easier to digest than formula. And because breastmilk contains a lower protein and mineral content, it makes a newborn's kidneys work less strenuously. The iron in breastmilk is more easily absorbed than that added to formula.

Ninety-nine percent of women who want to breast-feed are physically able to do so. The psychological condition of the mother, more often than her physical condition, is the key factor involved in successful breast-feeding. Breast-feeding is not automatic. It requires time, patience, understanding, and a sense of humor. It is a learning process for mother and baby alike. There are usually some problems during the first few weeks. This is especially true for women who have had a caesarean section or who are breast-feeding twins or a premature baby. But with proper guidance and support, these problems can be managed.

The greatest period of adjustment to breast-feeding occurs during the first seven to ten days after delivery. It is often helpful at this time to get information and guidance about breast-feeding from your hospital's nursing staff. If the nurses are unhelpful or if you want to talk with someone after you are home, call your local La Leche League chapter. This group was formed many years ago to promote breast-feeding. They should be listed in your phonebook.

Very useful advice and support can also be obtained from friends and relatives who have breast-fed. The more you know, the more comfortable you'll feel about breast-feeding and about advising other women who look to you for support.

Your Milk Supply

The amount of milk you produce depends on how much and how often your baby drinks. Sometimes, your milk production will lag behind your baby's appetite. It usually takes about forty-eight hours for breastmilk production to catch up with the increased demand brought on by an impending growth spurt.

You'll especially notice this lag when your baby is between fourteen and twenty-eight days old, a major hunger period for most infants. Many women become concerned at this time that they are not producing enough milk. But don't worry, your milk supply will increase after a day or two of frequent feedings. Do not supplement your baby's feedings with formula during this time. Supplemental bottle feeding will only decrease your production of breastmilk.

Can Breast-Fed Babies Be Overfed?

Breast-fed babies, like formula-fed ones, can be overfed. Such overfeeding usually results from nursing the baby for the wrong reason. Babies often receive comfort from sucking on a breast when they are tired, anxious, frustrated, or simply feeling the need to suck. Try a pacifier, some cuddling, a change of diapers, or a burping before you offer your breast to a baby who you suspect is not hungry.

Your Diet for Breast-Feeding

All the nutrients your baby needs can be found in your breastmilk —provided, of course, that you eat a balanced diet. When you're breast-feeding, your baby is still dependent on you for proper nourishment.

You'll need even more nutrients during breast-feeding than you did during pregnancy. This is because the baby you are nourishing is larger and growing more rapidly. It takes a newborn only four or five months to gain the same amount of weight he or she gained during nine months in the womb. To find out the amounts of each nutrient you need while breast-feeding, look at the "My Daily Vitamin and Mineral Needs" chart on pages 15-17.

Not all breastmilk is created equal. What you eat will make a difference. If your diet is low in nutrients, your breastmilk will be low in them, too. Also keep in mind that everything you eat or drink will likely appear in your breastmilk. For this reason, alcohol and caffeine should be consumed in moderation while breast-feeding. It is possible to give your child an unhealthy "caffeine high" or an equally unhealthy "alcohol low" by consuming too much of these substances. The commonly heard advice that a woman should relax with a beer or glass of wine before breast-feeding is not a good idea—for the baby or for the mother. If a woman were to drink alcohol before each feeding she would become more than relaxed. She would become drunk, for she would be downing about ten drinks a day during the early weeks of breast-feeding.

Over-the-counter and prescription drugs should be taken during breast-feeding only upon the advice of your health-care provider. They, too, can get into your breastmilk with possibly harmful consequences. Environmental contaminants such as PCB's and PBB's may appear in breastmilk if the mother has eaten contaminated food products. If you have reason to suspect that your breastmilk may contain any of these contaminants, try to have your milk analyzed. Your health-care provider may be able to help you have this done.

Raw Materials Needed for Breast-Feeding

During the first three months of breast-feeding, it takes about 800 calories a day to produce the amount of milk your baby needs. About

500 of these calories should come from your diet and the remainder from your stores of body fat.

Using up 300 calories from your fat stores each day will lead to a weight loss of about two-and-a-half pounds a month. After three months, breast-feeding will require about 1100 calories a day. As a result, you'll be losing even more weight. This will continue until your baby begins to eat solid foods in addition to breastmilk. Then your breastmilk production will level off or decrease.

Breast-feeding calories are, of course, in addition to the 2000 to 2200 daily calories you need to nourish your own body.

During breast-feeding, you also need to increase your protein intake by twenty grams a day to a total of sixty-four grams. Four daily servings of milk or milk products and two servings of meat or meat alternatives should supply the required level of protein.

You can meet your increased need for vitamins and minerals by daily eating two vitamin C-rich fruits or vegetables, a vitamin A-rich fruit or vegetable, two servings of other types of fruits and vegetables, and four servings of breads and cereals. One mineral may appear in small amounts in your breastmilk regardless of what you eat: fluoride. In areas where water is not fluoridated, fluoride supplements are often prescribed for babies before they are six months old.

In previous chapters, with the aid of a chart, you took a look at your diet to see how balanced it was before and during pregnancy. On pages 76 and 77 is a similar chart devised for breast-feeding mothers. Review your diet as you did before to make sure you have all your basic nutrition needs covered.

Foods That May Give Your Breast-Feeding Baby Gas

If you discover that your baby is experiencing considerable discomfort from intestinal gas, you may want to review your breast-feeding diet to see if any of the following items were on that day's menu: cabbage, cauliflower, broccoli, brussels sprouts, sauerkraut, onions, garlic, rhubarb, or curry. These foods contain substances that find their way into breastmilk. Babies sensitive to these substances will develop gas pains within hours of being breast-fed.

Try out these foods on your baby slowly. East small portions of them at first. Then wait and see if your baby reacts. If you are up at two o'clock in the morning comforting your baby who is having gas

How Balanced Is My Breast-Feeding Diet?

Food Group	Size of Standard Serving	Number of Servings I Had	Minimum Recommended Number of Servings	Difference between my Servings and Number Recommended
1. Dairy products			4	
milk	1 cup			
yogurt	1 cup			
cheese	1 1/2 ounce			
cottage cheese	1 cup			
2. Meat and meat alternates			2	
meat	3 ounces			
fish	3 ounces			
poultry	3 ounces			
dried beans	1 cup			
eggs	2			
peanut butter	4 tbsp			
peanuts, other nuts	1/2 cup or 3 ounces			
3. Vitamin A vegetables and fruits			1	
broccoli	1/2 cup			
carrots	1/2 cup			
collards	1/2 cup			
green peppers	1/2 cup			
spinach	1/2 cup			
sweet potato	1/2 cup			
winter squash	1/2 cup			
papaya	1 cup			
cataloupe	1/4 melon			
plums	1 cup			
apricots	3			
4. Vitamin C fruits and vegetables			2	
cataloupe	1 cup or 1/4 melon			
oranges/orange juice	1 or 6 ounces			
grapefruit/juice	1 or 6 ounces			
tomatoes/juice	1 or 1 cup			
strawberries	2/3 cup			
watermelon	1/2 cup			
papaya	1/2 cup			
broccoli	1/2 cup			
raw cabbage	1 cup			
green pepper	1/2 cup			
brussel sprouts	1/2 cup			
5. Other fruits and vegetables			2	
banana	1			
apples/juice	1 or 6 ounces			

How Balanced Is My Breast-Feeding Diet?—*Continued*

Food Group	Size of Standard Serving	Number of Servings I Had	Minimum Recommended Number of Servings	Difference between my Servings and Number Recommended
pears	1			
peaches	1			
grapes/juice	1/2 cup or 6 ounces			
potatoes	1 small or 1/2 cup			
corn	1/2 cup			
peas	1/2 cup			
beets	1/2 cup			
green beans	1/2 cup			
6. Breads and cereals			4	
bread	1 slice			
roll, biscuit, or				
muffin	1			
✓ tortilla	1			
ready-to-eat cereal	3/4 cup			
pasta	3/4 cup			
rice	3/4 cup			
7. "Miscellaneous"			2 or more depending on calorie need	
Butter, margarine, oil	1 tsp			
salad dressing	2 tbsp			
sour cream	1 tbsp			
cream cheese	1 tbsp			
mayonnaise	2 tsp			
gravy	1 tbsp			

pains, you should think seriously of giving up spicy foods or foods from the cabbage family while nursing.

Diet for the Breast-Feeding Vegetarian

Vegetarians who breast-feed their babies should take the same precautions that they did during pregnancy to ensure that their diets are rich in all necessary nutrients (see Chapter 3). For lacto-ovo vegetarians, this is easily done with a balanced diet. Take special care, however, to get enough protein, vitamin B_{12}, iron, zinc, and calcium. These nutrients, which are necessary for the production of breast-milk, are not present in large amounts in most fruits, vegetables, and grains.

The vegan diet requires more careful planning. It is much more difficult to ensure the health of a newborn on a vegan diet. Have a dietitian or nutritionist analyze your diet to make certain that you are receiving enough calories and protein, as well as the recommended RDA's of calcium, iron, zinc, vitamin B_{12}, vitamin D, iodine, and vitamin B_6. The recommended RDA's for breast-feeding mothers appear on the "My Daily Vitamin and Mineral Needs" chart on pages 15-17.

Postscript

Farewell readers of this book. You have taken the time and effort to give yourself and your baby a priceless gift—the nutritional advantage. May you live in health and one day you see your children's children begin life with the same wonderful advantage.

Appendix

A BALANCED SEVEN-DAY MENU PLAN
FOR PREGNANCY

Day One — Sunday

Breakfast

Orange juice, 6 oz
pancakes, 3, with
maple syrup, 2 tbsp
and margarine, 1 tbsp
skim milk, 1 cup

Lunch

chili con carne, 1 cup
hard roll, 1
margarine, 1 tbsp
skim milk, 1 cup

Supper

spinach salad, 1 cup
with Italian dressing, 2 tbsp
pot roast, 4 oz
noodles, 3/4 cup
gravy, 3 tbsp
green beans, 1/2 cup
skim milk, 1 cup

Snacks

popcorn, 2 cups
apple, 1
cheddar cheese, 2 oz

Nutrient Analysis[a]

nutrient	amount	% of RDA
calories	2318 kcal	101
protein	116 g	156
calcium	1730 mg	144
iron[b]	20.4 mg	113
Vitamin A	7195 IU	144
Thiamin	1.7 mg	121
Riboflavin	2.7 mg	177
Niacin	21.8 mg	145
Vitamin C	125 mg	157

[a]Nutrient analyses provided by Nutrition Support Headquarters, Inc., Minneapolis, Minnesota.

[b]For these calculations, a RDA for iron of 18 mg is used. It is recommended that pregnant women take 30-60 mg of iron as a supplement in the last half of pregnancy.

**A BALANCED SEVEN-DAY MENU PLAN
FOR PREGNANCY** —*Continued*

Day Two—Monday

Breakfast
cantaloupe, 1/4 melon
corn flakes, 1 cup
with sugar, 2 tsp
and milk, 1 cup
Lunch
tomato soup, 1 cup
tuna-salad sandwich
on whole-wheat bread
skim milk, 1 cup
Supper
baked chicken, 4 oz
baked beans, 3/4 cup
broccoli spears, 1 cup
dinner rolls, 1
margarine, 2 tsp
skim milk, 1 cup
Snacks
bagel, 1
with cream cheese, 1 tbsp
orange, 1

Nutrient Analysis[a]

nutrient	amount	% of RDA
calories	1971 kcal	86
protein	122 g	165
calcium	1140 mg	95
iron	17.9 mg	100
Vitamin A	4781 IU	96
Thiamin	1.67 mg	119
Riboflavin	2.16 mg	144
Niacin	36 mg	240
Vitamin C	335 mg	423

**A BALANCED SEVEN-DAY MENU PLAN
FOR PREGNANCY** —*Continued*

Day Three — Tuesday

Breakfast

strawberries, 1/2 cup
bran muffins, 2
with margarine, 1 tbsp
skim milk, 1 cup

Lunch

pizza with cheese and sausage, 3 slices
lemonade, 12 oz

Supper

tossed salad, 1 cup
oil and vinegar dressing, 2 tbsp.
sauteed calf liver, 3 oz
with bacon, 2 strips
and onions, 1/8 cup
peas, 1/2 cup
whole-wheat rolls, 2
ice cream, 1 cup
skim milk, 1 cup

Snacks

graham crackers, 4
milk, 1 cup

Nutrient Analysis[a]

nutrient	amount	% of RDA
calories	2256 kcal	98
protein	110 g	149
calcium	1229 mg	102
iron	18.7 mg	104
Vitamin A	37,164 IU	743
Thiamin	1.68 mg	120
Riboflavin	6.69 mg	446
Niacin	27.6 mg	184
Vitamin C	180 mg	225

**A BALANCED SEVEN-DAY MENU PLAN
FOR PREGNANCY** —*Continued*

Day Four—Wednesday

Breakfast
apple juice, 6 oz
oatmeal, 3/4 cup
with brown sugar, 2 tbsp
and half-and-half, 1/4 cup

Lunch
split pea soup, 1 cup
macaroni and cheese, 1 cup
spinach, 1/2 cup
skim milk, 1 cup

Supper
ground-beef pattie, 3 oz
zucchini, 1/2 cup
corn, 1/2 cup
french bread, 1 piece
margarine, 2 tsp
pudding, 1 cup
skim milk, 1 cup

Snacks
orange, 1
cake, 1 piece
skim milk, 1 cup

Nutrient Analysis[a]

nutrient	amount	% of RDA
calories	2075 kcal	90
protein	101 g	136
calcium	1870 mg	156
iron	15.7 mg	87
Vitamin A	13,095 IU	262
Thiamin	1.54 mg	110
Riboflavin	3.17 mg	211
Niacin	15.8 mg	105
Vitamin C	135 mg	168

A BALANCED SEVEN-DAY MENU PLAN
FOR PREGNANCY—*Continued*

Day Five—Thursday

Breakfast

grapefruit, 1/2
bran flakes, 1 cup
with sliced peaches, 1/4 cup
and skim milk, 1 cup

Lunch

turkey, 3 oz
on whole-wheat bread, 2 slices
with lettuce, 1 large leaf,
tomato, 3 slices
and mayonnaise, 1 tbsp
dill pickle, 1
tea, 1 cup

Supper

antipasto salad, 1 cup
(lettuce, 1/2 cup; tomato, 1/8 cup;
green olives, 1 oz; ham, 1 oz)
spaghetti with meatballs, 1½ cups
Italian bread, 2 slices
butter, 2 tsp
skim milk, 1 cup

Snacks

banana, 1
skim milk, 1 cup

Nutrient Analysis[a]

nutrient	amount	% of RDA
calories	2000 kcal	87
protein	98 g	132
calcium	1200 mg	100
iron	26 mg	144
Vitamin A	4,100 IU	82
Thiamin	1.6 mg	114
Riboflavin	2.6 mg	173
Niacin	2.6 mg	173
Vitamin C	110 mg	138

**A BALANCED SEVEN-DAY MENU PLAN
FOR PREGNANCY** —*Continued*

Day Six — Friday

Breakfast

grape juice, 6 oz
whole-wheat toast, 2 slices
with melted American cheese, 2 oz
skim milk, 1 cup

Lunch

sliced tomato, 1/2 cup
with oil, 1 tbsp, and
vinegar, 1 tsp. dressing
cottage cheese, 1/2 cup
with fruit cocktail, 3/4 cup
saltine crackers, 6
lemonade, 8 oz

Supper

egg rolls, 2
sweet and sour pork, 4 oz
rice, 3/4 cup
almond cookies, 2
tea, 1 cup

Snacks

raisins, 1/4 cup
peanuts, 1/8 cup
orange juice, 6 oz

Nutrient Analysis[a]

nutrient	amount	% of RDA
calories	2300 kcal	100
protein	90 g	122
calcium	1200 mg	100
iron	12 mg	67
Vitamin A	2800 IU	56
Thiamin	1.5 mg	107
Riboflavin	1.7 mg	113
Niacin	16 mg	107
Vitamin C	140 mg	175

A BALANCED SEVEN-DAY MENU PLAN
FOR PREGNANCY —*Continued*

Day Seven—Saturday

Breakfast
orange juice, 6 oz
cheese omelet, with eggs, 2
and cheese, 1 oz
and whole-wheat toast, 2 slices
margarine, 2 tsp
skim milk, 1 cup
Lunch
hamburger, 3 oz
with cheese, 1 oz
on bun, 1
cole slaw, 1/2 cup
yogurt, 1 cup with
peaches, 1/2 cup
lemonade, 12 oz
Supper
bean soup, 1 cup
roast pork, 3 oz
mashed potatoes, 1/2 cup
carrots, 1/2 cup
margarine, 1 tsp
fruit pie, 1 piece
skim milk, 1 cup
Snacks
applesauce, 1/2 cup

Nutrient Analysis

nutrient	amount	% of RDA
calories	2600 kcal	113
protein	120 g	162
calcium	1600 mg	133
iron	15 mg	83
Vitamin A	12,000 IU	240
Thiamin	2.0 mg	143
Riboflavin	2.5 mg	143
Niacin	17 mg	167
Vitamin C	190 mg	238

Nutrient Analysis
Summary for the Seven-Day Menu

nutrient	amount	% of RDA
calories	2217	96
protein	108	146
calcium	1424	119
iron	18	100
Vitamin A	11,591	232
Thiamin	1.67	119
Riboflavin	3.1	207
Niacin	22.9	153
Vitamin C	174	218

CALORIC VALUES OF FOODS WITHIN FOOD GROUPS[a]

Milk and Dairy Products

Food; Amount	Calories
evaporated milk; 1 cup	345
custard; 1 cup	305
ice cream; 1 cup	290
ice milk; 1 cup	285
soft serve; 1 cup	265
cottage cheese; 1 cup	260
cocoa; 1 cup	245
pudding; 1 cup	225
cottage cheese, low fat; 1 cup	170
milk, whole; 1 cup	160
milk, 2%; 1 cup	145
yogurt, low fat; 1 cup	120
swiss cheese; 1 ounce	105
cheddar cheese; 1 ounce	105
blue cheese; 1 ounce	105
American cheese; 1 ounce	105
skim milk; 1 cup	90

Meat and Meat Alternatives

Food; Amount	Calories
chili; 1 cup	335
spaghetti with meat sauce; 1 cup	330
ham; 3 ounces	245
hamburger, regular; 3 ounces	245
roast beef, lean; 3 ounces	245
sausage links; 3 ounces	245
roast lamb, lean; 3 ounces	235
dried beans, cooked; 1 cup	230
steak, lean; 3 ounces	220
stew; 1 cup	216
almonds; 1/4 cup	213
peanuts; 1/4 cup	210
walnuts; 1/4 cup	198
cashews; 1/4 cup	196
corned beef; 3 ounces	185
hamburger, lean; 3 ounces	185
cheese pizza; 1 piece	185
veal cutlet; 3 ounces	185
pork roast; 3 ounces	175
beef liver; 3 ounces	173
tuna; 3 ounces	170
hot dog; 1	155
haddock, fried; 3 ounces	140
pork chop, lean; 3 ounces	135
chicken, baked, no skin; 3 ounces	115
shrimp; 3 ounces	100
peanut butter; 1 tablespoon	95
egg; 1	80
bologna; 2 slices	80

[a]Information provided by Nutrition Support Hdqtrs., Minneapolis, MN.

CALORIC VALUES OF FOODS
WITHIN FOOD GROUPS—*Continued*
Vitamin A Fruits and Vegetables

Food; Amount	Calories
peaches, sliced; 1 cup	225
apricots, canned; 1 cup	220
plums, canned; 1 cup	220
sweet potatoes, boiled; 1	170
winter squash; 1 cup	130
watermelon; 2 cups	110
apricots, dried; 1/4 cup	98
vegetable-beef soup; 1 cup	80
papaya; 1 cup	70
collards; 1 cup	55
brussel sprouts; 1 cup	55
apricots, raw; 3	50
tomatoes, canned; 1 cup	50
cantaloupe; 1/2 melon	50
carrots, cooked; 1 cup	45
tomato juice; 1 cup	44
broccoli; 1 cup	40
spinach; 1 cup	40
carrots, raw; 1	20

Vitamin C Fruits and Vegetables

Food; Amount	Calories
cranberry juice cocktail; 1 cup	165
broccoli; 1 cup	140
tangerine juice; 1 cup	125
orange juice; 1 cup	120
grapefruit juice; 1 cup	95
papaya; 1 cup	70
orange; 1 medium	65
cantaloupe; 1/2 melon	60
collards; 1 cup	55
brussel sprouts; 1 cup	55
strawberries, raw; 1 cup	55
grapefruit; 1/2	45
tomato; 1 medium	40
spinach; 1 cup	40
cabbage, cooked; 1 cup	30
cauliflower, cooked; 1 cup	25
cabbage, raw; 1 cup	20
green pepper, raw; 1/2	8
lemon; 1/4	5

Other Fruits and Vegetables

Food; Amount	Calories
rhubarb, cooked, sweetened; 1 cup	385
applesauce; 1 cup	230
plums, canned; 1 cup	205
prune juice; 1 cup	200
peaches, canned; 1 cup	200

CALORIC VALUES OF FOODS
WITHIN FOOD GROUPS—*Continued*

Other Fruits and Vegetables

Food; Amount	Calories
pears, canned; 1 cup	195
fruit cocktail, canned; 1 cup	195
pineapple, canned; 1 cup	195
avocado; 1/2	190
lima beans; 1 cup	180
corn; 1 cup	170
grape juice; 1 cup	135
pineapple juice; 1 cup	135
apple juice; 1 cup	120
raisins; 1/4 cup	120
green peas; 1 cup	115
watermelon; 1 wedge	115
banana; 1	100
pear; 1	100
potato, baked; 1 medium	90
blueberries; 1 cup	85
pineapple, raw; 1 cup	75
prunes, uncooked; 4	70
raspberries; 1 cup	70
apple; 1 medium	70
grapes; 1 cup	65
beets; 1 cup	55
tangerine; 1 medium	40
peach; 1 medium	35
bean sprouts; 1 cup	35
asparagus; 1 cup	30
green beans; 1 cup	30
summer squash; 1 cup	30
plum; 1 medium	25
mushrooms; 1/4 cup	10
lettuce; 1/8 head	8
cucumbers; 6 slices	5
celery; 1 stalk	5

Breads and Cereals

Food; Amount	Calories
Danish pastry; 1	275
rice; 1 cup	225
waffle; 1	205
noodles; 1 cup	200
bagel; 1	165
macaroni; 1 cup	155
hard roll; 1	155
spaghetti; 1 cup	155
oatmeal; 1 cup	130
grits; 1 cup	125

CALORIC VALUES OF FOODS
WITHIN FOOD GROUPS—*Continued*

Breads and Cereals

Food; Amount	Calories
doughnut; 1	125
muffin; 1	120
farina; 1 cup	105
bran flakes; 1 cup	105
biscuit; 1	105
corn flakes; 1 cup	100
Italian bread; 1 slice (1 oz)	78
white bread; 1 slice	70
whole-wheat bread; 1 slice	65
rye bread; 1 slice	60
pancake; 1	60
crackers; 4 saltines	50
French bread; 1 slice (1/2 oz)	41

Miscellaneous Foods

Food; Amount	Calories
oil (all types); 1 tablespoon	125
cream cheese; 2 tablespoons	107
mayonnaise; 1 tablespoon	100
bacon; 2 slices	86
Russian dressing; 1 tablespoon	80
blue-cheese dressing; 1 tablespoon	75
French dressing; 1 tablespoon	65
whipped cream; 2 tablespoons	55
margarine; 1 teaspoon	35
butter; 1 teaspoon	35
tartar sauce; 1 tablespoon	34
half-and-half; 1 tablespoon	22
sour cream; 1 tablespoon	20

FOOD SOURCES OF KEY NUTRIENTS[a]

Protein

Food; Amount	G. Protein
cottage cheese, lowfat; 1 cup	28
chicken, no skin; 3 ounces	27
roast beef; 3 ounces	25
pork chop, lean; 3 ounces	25
tuna; 3 ounces	24
steak, lean; 3 ounces	24
veal cutlet; 3 ounces	23
lamb, roast; 3 ounces	22
beef liver; 3 ounces	22
shrimp; 3 ounces	21
hamburger, regular; 3 ounces	21
haddock, fried; 3 ounces	19

[a]Information provided by Nutrition Support, Inc., Minneapolis, MN.

FOOD SOURCES OF KEY NUTRIENTS —*Continued*

Protein

Food; Amount	G. Protein
ham; 3 ounces	18
sausage links; 3 ounces	17
beans, dried, cooked; 1 cup	15
stew; 1 cup	15
custard; 1 cup	13
lima beans; 1 cup	12
yogurt, lowfat; 1 cup	12
peanuts; 1/4 cup	9
whole milk; 1 cup	8
cheddar cheese; 3 ounces	7
egg; 1	6
peanut butter; 1 tablespoon	4

Total Fat

Food; Amount	G. Fat
spare ribs; 3	35.0
prime rib; 3 ounces	33.5
lamb chop; 3 ounces	28.0
sirloin steak; 3 ounces	27.0
soufflé; 1 cup	25.7
chicken pot pie; 1.5 cups	25.4
hash; 1 cup	25.0
pork roast; 3 ounces	24.0
tamales; 2	23.7
knockwurst; 3.5 ounces	23.2
macaroni anc cheese; 1 cup	22.0
sweet 'n sour pork; 1.5 cups	21.7
sesame seeds; 1/4 cup	20.0
Hollandaise sauce; 1/4 cup	18.5
pecan pie; 1 piece	18.3
avocado; 1/2 (1/2 cup)	18.0
cream pie; 1 piece	18.0
walnuts; 1 ounce (14 halves)	17.8
tostada; 1	17.6
fruit pie; 1 piece	17.5
egg foo young; 1 cup	17.4
sunflower seeds; 1/4 cup	17.0
tongue; 3.5 ounces	17.0
chuck roast; 3 ounces	16.5
hamburger, regular; 3 ounces	16.5
chili; 1 cup	15.5
Danish pastry; 1	15.5
chocolate eclair; 1	15.4
oil (all types); 1 tablespoon	15.0
gravy; 1/4 cup	14.0
peanuts; 1 ounce (30 nuts)	13.9
round steak; 3 ounces	13.0

FOOD SOURCES OF KEY NUTRIENTS – *Continued*

Total Fat

Food; Amount	G. Fat
bacon; 2 slices	12.5
cheese cake; 3 ounces (1/2 cup)	12.5
mayonnaise; 1 tablespoon	12.0
pork sausage; 2 links	11.3
heavy cream; 2 tablespoons	11.3
cheddar cheese; 1 ounce	11.3
salami; 1 ounce	11.0
doughnut; 1	11.0
beef stew; 1 cup	10.5

Saturated Fats (SF)

Food; Amount	G. SF
Hollandaise sauce; 1/4 cup	23.0
lamb chop; 3 ounces	18.0
banana split; 2 cups	9.0
sirloin steak; 3 ounces	9.0
coconut; 1 ounce	9.0
ice cream; 1 cup	8.8
hamburger, regular; 3 ounces	8.0
custard; 1 cup	7.8
heavy cream; 2 tablespoons	7.0
milkshake; 12 ounces	7.0
cheddar cheese; 1 ounce	5.7
milk, whole; 1 cup	5.3
blue cheese; 1 ounce	5.3
yogurt, plain; 1 cup	5.3
Edam cheese; 1 ounce	5.1
brick cheese; 1 ounce	5.0
American cheese; 1 ounce	5.0
cottage cheese, creamed; 1 cup	4.8
mozzarella cheese; 1 ounce	4.7
white sauce; 1/4 cup	4.4
bacon; 2 slices	4.0
sour cream; 2 tablespoons	3.5
chicken breast; 3 ounces	3.0
milk, 2%; 1 cup	2.9
cashews; 1 ounce (15 nuts)	2.8
peanuts; 1 ounce (30 nuts)	2.6
butter; 1 teaspoon	2.5
walnuts; 1 ounce (14 halves)	2.1
cottage cheese, lowfat, 1 cup	2.0

Polyunsaturated Fats (PUF)

Food; Amount	G. PUF
pecans; 1 ounce (20 halves)	17.7
turkey pot pie; 1.5 cups	16.0
beef pot pie; 1.5 cups	15.0
Brazil nuts; 1 ounce (6 nuts)	14.7

FOOD SOURCES OF KEY NUTRIENTS—*Continued*
Polyunsaturated Fats (PUF)

Food; Amount	G. PUF
almonds; 1 ounce (14 nuts)	14.0
chicken pot pie; 1.5 cups	14.0
olive oil; 1 tablespoon	12.0
soybean oil; 1 tablespoon	11.0
walnuts; 1 ounce (14 halves)	10.5
cashews; 1 ounce (15 nuts)	10.1
sesame seeds; 1/4 cup	10.0
peanuts; 1 ounce (30 nuts)	10.0
avocado; 1/2 piece (1/2 cup)	9.0
mayonnaise; 1 tablespoon	9.0
Italian dressing; 1 tablespoon	7.0
chicken breast; 3 ounces	7.0
soybeans; 1 cup	6.0
fried bread; 2 ounces (1/4 cup)	6.0
blue cheese; 1 ounce	5.0
French dressing; 1 tablespoon	4.2
turkey, dark meat; 3 ounces	4.0
chicken thigh; 2 ounces	4.0
tofu; 1/2 cup	3.6

Cholesterol

Food; Amount	Mg. Cholesterol
chicken liver; 3 ounces	522
Hollandaise sauce; 1/4 cup	382
pork, fat untrimmed; 3 ounces	340
egg foo young; 1 cup	280
beef liver; 3 ounces	255
egg; 1	252
soufflé; 1 cup	251
custard; 1 cup	240
oysters; 6	230
veal parmagiani; 1 cup	206
lobster; 3.5 ounces	200
banana split; 2 cups	180
pumpkin pie; 1 piece	150
tongue; 3.5 ounces	140
shrimp; 3 ounces	126
corned beef; 3 ounces	120
pecan pie; 1 piece	92
crab; 3 ounces	84
turkey, dark meat; 3 ounces	84
lamb, lean; 3 ounces	84
veal, lean; 3 ounces	83
chocolate eclair; 1	80
pork, fat trimmed; 3 ounces	74
chicken, with skin; 3 ounces	74
chicken, without skin; 3 ounces	71

FOOD SOURCES OF KEY NUTRIENTS—*Continued*

Cholesterol

Food; Amount	Mg. Cholesterol
hamburger, regular; 3 ounces	60
turkey, light meat; 3 ounces	65
sausage; 3 ounces	55
beef, fat trimmed; 3 ounces	50
hamburger, lean; 3 ounces	50
heavy cream; 2 tablespoons	40
yogurt, plain; 1 cup	34
milk, whole; 1 cup	34
ice cream, vanilla; 1/2 cup	33
Edam cheese; 1 ounce	29
mozzarella cheese; 1 ounce	27
cheddar cheese; 1 ounce	26
brick cheese	25
American cheese; 1 ounce	25
blue cheese; 1 ounce	24
milk, 2%; 1 cup	22
cottage cheese, creamed; 1/2 cup	21
sour cream; 2 tablespoons	20
half and half; 2 tablespoons	13
butter; 1 teaspoon	13
mayonnaise; 1 tablespoon	11
cottage cheese, low fat; 1/2 cup	8
skim milk; 1 cup	7

Carbohydrates

Food; Amount	G. Carbohydrate
rice; 1 cup	50
corn; 1 cup	40
sweet potato, boiled; 1 medium	39
beans; 1 cup	38
noodles; 1 cup	37
lima beans; 1 cup	34
winter squash; 1 cup	32
macaroni; 1 cup	32
spaghetti; 1 cup	32
bagel; 1	30
hard roll; 1	30
bran flakes; 1 cup	28
grits; 1 cup	27
potatoes, mashed; 1 cup	25
wheat flakes; 1 cup	24
parsnips; 1 cup	23
oatmeal; 1 cup	23
farina; 1 cup	22
potato, baked; 1 medium	21
corn flakes; 1 cup	21
French fries; 10 pieces	20

FOOD SOURCES OF KEY NUTRIENTS—*Continued*
Carbohydrates

Food; Amount	G. Carbohydrate
green peas; 1 cup	19
muffin; 1	17
Italian bread; 1 slice	16
dinner roll; 1	15
whole-wheat bread; 1 slice	14
white bread; 1 slice	13
rye bread; 1 slice	13
crackers; 4 saltines	8
French bread; 1 slice (1/2 oz)	8

Sucrose

Food; Amount	G. Sucrose
banana split; 2 cups	91.8
sherbert; 1 cup	56.8
fruit, canned in syrup; 1 cup	20-56
soft drinks; 12 ounces	27-43
presweetened cereals; 1 cup	28-40
milkshake; 12 ounces	33.8
applesauce; 1 cup	32.8
fruit-flavored drinks; 1 cup	31.5
yogurt with fruit; 1 cup	31.5
hard candy; 1 ounce	30.0
popsicle; 1	28.4
sweet 'n sour pork; 1.5 cups	24.0
pumpkin pie; 1 piece	22.6
cake with icing; 1 piece (1/2 cup)	21.0
fudge; 1 oz	20.0
instant breakfast; 1 cup	19.0
cream pie; 1 piece	18.0
fruit pie; 1 piece	17.4
chocolate sauce; 2 tablespoons	17.2
carmels; 3 squares	16.0
coffee cake; 1 piece (1/2 cup)	14.3
sweet pickle; 1 (1/8 cup)	12.0
milk chocolate; 1 oz	12.0
maple syrup; 1 tablespoon	12.0
brownie; 1 piece (1/4 cup)	11.1
peas, canned; 1 cup	10.8
molasses; 1 tablespoon	10.7
jam, jelly; 1 teaspoon	10.6
cranberry jelly; 1/8 cup	9.3
chocolate milk; 1 cup	8.6
cookies; 1	7.5
Danish pastry; 1 piece	7.4
doughnut; 1	6.0
white sugar; 1 teaspoon	5.0
graham crackers; 1	3.4

FOOD SOURCES OF KEY NUTRIENTS—*Continued*

Fiber

Food	G. Fiber
All Bran; 1 ounce (1/3 cup)	9.0
Bran Buds; 1 cup	6.0
bran; 1/4 cup	4.2
blackberries; 1 cup	4.0
raspberries: 1 cup	4.0
green peas, canned; 1 cup	4.0
strawberries; 1 cup	4.0
pork 'n beans; 1 cup	3.4
green peas, frozen: 1 cup	3.2
black-eyed peas; 1 cup	3.0
bran muffin; 1	3.0
lentil beans; 1 cup	3.0
blueberries; 1 cup	3.0
white beans: 1 cup	3.0
sunflower seeds; 1/4 cup	2.0
mixed vegetables; 1 cup	2.0
chef's salad; 2 cups	2.0
broccoli; 1 cup	1.8
Raisin Bran; 1 cup	1.7
rutabagas; 1 cup	1.6
collard greens: 1 cup	1.6
carrots, raw or cooked: 1 cup	1.6
apple; 1 medium	1.5
watermelon; 2 cups	1.5
tomato; 1 medium	1.4
corn; 1 cup	1.4
Bran Chex; 2/3 cup	1.3
sweet potato; 1 medium (3/4 cup)	1.3
Bran Flakes; 1 cup	1.3
banked potato; 3/4 cup	1.2
coconut; 1/8 cup	1.2
pear; 1 medium	1.0
mango; 1 medium	1.0
apricots, dried; 3 pieces	1.0
Country Morning: 1 cup	0.9
green pepper; 1/2 cup	0.9
orange: 1 medium	0.8
peach; 1 medium	0.8
dates; 1/3 cup (10 pieces)	0.8
tossed salad; 1/4 cup	0.8
banana; 1 medium	0.8
tomato juice; 3/4 cup	0.7

Niacin

Food; Amount	Mg. Niacin
beef liver; 3 ounces	12.5
tuna; 3 ounces	10.1
chicken; 3 ounces	7.4

FOOD SOURCES OF KEY NUTRIENTS — *Continued*

Niacin

Food; Amount	Mg. Niacin
salmon; 3 ounces	6.8
veal roast; 3 ounces	6.6
peanuts; 1/4 cup	6.2
steak; 3 ounces	4.8
pork roast; 3 ounces	4.7
lamb roast; 3 ounces	4.7
veal cutlet; 3 ounces	4.6
stew; 1 cup	4.4
pork chop; 3 ounces	3.8
green peas; 1 cup	3.7
roast beef; 3 ounces	3.1
Brewer's yeast; 1 tablespoon	3.0
haddock; 3 ounces	2.7
collards; 1 cup	2.4
corn; 1 cup	2.3
lima beans; 1 cup	2.2
beer; 12 ounces	2.2
bran flakes; 1 cup	2.2
avocado; 1/2 piece (1/2 cup)	2.1
mashed potatoes; 1 cup	2.0
asparagus; 1 cup	2.0
noodles; 1 cup	1.9
French fries; 10 pieces	1.8
macaroni and cheese; 1 cup	1.8
baked potato; 1 medium	1.7
summer squash; 1 cup	1.6
peaches, canned; 1 cup	1.6
macaroni; 1 cup	1.5
spaghetti; 1 cup	1.5

Vitamin A

Food; Amount	Mg. Vitamin A
beef liver; 3 ounces	45,420
carrots; 1 cup	15,220
pumpkin, canned; 1 cup	14,590
spinach, cooked; 1 cup	14,580
sweet potato; 1 medium	11,610
collards; 1 cup	10,260
winter squash; 1 cup	8,610
turnip greens, cooked; 1 cup	8,270
kale, cooked; 1 cup	8,140
beet greens, cooked; 1 cup	7,400
cantaloupe; 1/2 melon	6,540
broccoli; 1 cup	3,880
papaya; 1 cup	3,190
plums, canned; 1 cup	2,970

FOOD SOURCES OF KEY NUTRIENTS — *Continued*

Vitamin A

Food; Amount	Mg. Vitamin A
vegetable soup; 1 cup	2,940
apricots, raw; 3	2,890
vegetable-beef soup; 1 cup	2,700
watermelon; 2 cups	2,510
apricot nectar; 1 cup	2,380
peaches, sliced; 1 cup	2,230
tomatoes, canned; 1 cup	2,170
tomato juice; 1 cup	1,940
tomato, raw; 1 medium	1,640
peach, raw; 1 medium	1,320
asparagus; 1 cup	1,310

Vitamin B_6

Food; Amount	Mg. Vitamin B_6
turnip greens; 1 cup	1.4
brussel sprouts; 1 cup	0.8
pork 'n beans; 1 cup	0.8
kidney beans; 1 cup	0.8
mackerel; 3.5 ounces	0.7
beef liver; 3 ounces	0.7
oysters; 1/2 cup	0.6
chicken breast; 1	0.6
black-eyed peas; 1 cup	0.6
banana; 1 medium	0.6
bean soup; 1 cup	0.5
chicken liver; 2.5 ounces	0.5
baked potato; 1 medium	0.5
tomato juice; 1 cup	0.4
chicken thigh; 1	0.4
asparagus; 1 cup	0.4
avocado; 1/2 (1/2 cup)	0.4
hamburger, regular; 3 ounces	0.4
hamburger, lean; 3 ounces	0.4
spinach, cooked; 1 cup	0.4
sunflower seeds; 1/4 cup	0.4
sirloin steak; 3 ounces	0.3
chuck roast; 3 ounces	0.3
prime rib; 3 ounces	0.3
cod; 4 ounces	0.3
crab; 3.5 ounces	0.3
artichoke; 1	0.3
turkey, dark meat; 3 ounces	0.3
veal cutlet; 3 ounces	0.3
wheat germ; 1/4 cup	0.3
salmon; 3.5 ounces	0.3
pork roast; 3 ounces	0.3

FOOD SOURCES OF KEY NUTRIENTS — *Continued*

Vitamin B_{12}

Food; Amount	Mcg. B_{12}
beef liver; 3 ounces	68.0
oysters; 1/2 cup	21.6
clams; 1/2 cup	20.0
chicken liver; 2.5 ounces	17.5
mackerel; 3.5 ounces	9.4
salmon; 3.7 ounces	7.6
Tuna Helper; 1 cup	4.4
liverwurst; 1 ounce	4.2
tuna salad; 1/2 cup	2.2
round steak; 3 ounces	2.2
tuna; 3.3 ounces	2.2
stew; 1 cup	1.6
prime rib; 3 ounces	1.5
sirloin steak; 3 ounces	1.5
chuck roast; 3 ounces	1.5
lamb, lean; 3 ounces	1.5
hamburger, regular; 3 ounces	1.5
corned beef; 3 ounces	1.5
meatballs; 2 (1/2 cup)	1.5
scallops; 3.5 ounces	1.1

Riboflavin

Food; Amount	Mg. Riboflavin
beef liver; 3 ounces	3.20
milk, 2%; 1 cup	0.52
custard; 1 cup	0.50
milk, skim; 1 cup	0.44
yogurt, low fat; 1 cup	0.44
milk, whole, 1 cup	0.41
macaroni and cheese; 1 cup	0.40
collards; 1 cup	0.37
pudding; 1 cup	0.36
Brewer's yeast; 1 tablespoon	0.34
winter squash; 1 cup	0.27
asparagus; 1 cup	0.26
avocado; 1/2 piece (1/2 cup)	0.26
veal roast; 3 ounces	0.26
spinach, cooked; 1 cup	0.25
lamb roast; 3 ounces	0.23
pork roast; 3 ounces	0.22
brussel sprouts; 1 cup	0.22
veal cutlet; 3 ounces	0.21
steak; 3 ounces	0.19
pork chop; 3 ounces	0.18
hamburger, regular; 3 ounces	0.18
green peas; 1 cup	0.17
stew; 1 cup	0.17

FOOD SOURCES OF KEY NUTRIENTS —*Continued*

Riboflavin

Food; Amount	Mg. Riboflavin
lima beans; 1 cup	0.17
summer squash, 1 cup	0.16
chicken; 3 ounces	0.16

Thiamin

Food; Amount	Mg. Thiamin
pork roast; 3 ounces	0.78
sunflower seeds, 1/4 cup	0.70
pork chop; 3.5 ounces	0.63
green peas; 1 cup	0.44
black-eyed peas; 1 cup	0.41
collards; 1 cup	0.27
limas beans; 1 cup	0.25
beans; 1 cup	0.25
chicken pot pie; 1.5 cups	0.25
beef pot pie; 1.5 cups	0.25
rice; 1 cup	0.23
beef liver; 3 ounces	0.23
asparagus; 1 cup	0.23
orange juice; 1 cup	0.22
noodles; 1 cup	0.22
pork sausage; 2 links	0.21
macaroni; 1 cup	0.20
spaghetti; 1 cup	0.20
oatmeal; 1 cup	0.19
avocado; 1/2 piece (1/2 cup)	0.15
broccoli; 1 cup	0.14
lamb chop; 4 ounces	0.14

Calcium

Food; Amount	Mg. Calcium
evaporated milk; 1 cup	635
sardines; 3 ounces	372
milk, 2%; 1 cup	352
milk, skim; 1 cup	296
cocoa; 1 cup	295
yogurt, low fat; 1 cup	294
collards; 1 cup	289
milk, whole; 1 cup	288
soft serve; 1 cup	273
yogurt, regular; 1 cup	272
Swiss cheese; 1 ounce	262
cabbage, raw; 1 cup	252
dandelion greens; 1 cup	252
turnip greens; 1 cup	252
pudding; 1 cup	250
cream soup; 1 cup	240

FOOD SOURCES OF KEY NUTRIENTS—*Continued*
Calcium

Food; Amount	Mg. Calcium
cottage cheese, creamed; 1 cup	230
oysters; 1 cup	226
cheddar cheese; 1 ounce	213
spinach, cooked; 1 cup	212
rhubarb; 1 cup	212
ice milk; 1 cup	204
macaroni and cheese; 1 cup	199
American cheese; 1 ounce	198
ice cream; 1 cup	194
cottage cheese, low fat; 1 cup	180

Panthothenic Acid (PA)

Food; Amount	Mg. PA
beef liver; 3 ounces	6.5
chicken liver; 2.5 ounces	4.2
brussel sprouts; 1 cup	2.2
custard; 1 cup	1.8
leeks; 1 cup	1.6
yogurt, lowfat; 1 cup	1.3
hash; 1 cup	1.2
black-eyed peas; 1 cup	1.2
asparagus; 1 cup	1.2
chow mein; 1 cup	1.2
watermelon; 2 cups	1.2
split peas; 1 cup	1.2
avocado; 1/2 (1/2 cup)	1.1
cauliflower, raw; 1 cup	1.0
veal steak; 3.5 ounces	1.0
turkey, dark meat; 3 ounces	1.0
sweet potato; 1 medium	1.0
egg; 1	0.9
yogurt, regular; 1 cup	0.9
mackerel; 3.5 ounces	0.9
milk, 2%; 1 cup	0.9
milk, skim; 1 cup	0.8
milk, whole; 1 cup	0.8
flounder; 3.5 ounces	0.8
sole; 3.5 ounces	0.8
honeydew melon; 1/4 melon	0.8
pork roast; 3 ounces	0.8
cantaloupe; 1/2 melon	0.8
baked potato; 1 medium	0.8
veal cutlet; 3 ounces	0.8
chicken breast; 1	0.8
mushrooms; 1/2 cup	0.8
liverwurst; 1 ounce	0.8
broccoli, 1 cup	0.8

FOOD SOURCES OF KEY NUTRIENTS —*Continued*

Zinc

Food; Amount	Mg. Zinc
oysters; 6	50.0
black-eyed peas; 1 cup	9.0
crab; 3.5 ounces (1/2 cup)	8.0
Instant Breakfast; 1 cup	5.8
chick peas; 1 cup	5.4
steak, lean; 3 ounces	5.0
hamburger, lean; 3 ounces	4.9
veal parmiginai; 7.5 ounces	4.6
Quarter Pounder; 1	4.6
beef liver; 3 ounces	4.3
chili; 1 cup	4.2
veal cutlet; 3 ounces	4.1
egg roll; 1	4.0
turkey, dark meat; 3 ounces	3.7
chuck roast; 3 ounces	3.7
hamburger, regular; 3 ounces	3.7
Big Mac; 1	3.7
Whopper; 1	3.7
lamb; 3 ounces	3.6
ham; 3 ounces	3.4
prime rib; 3 ounces	3.1
meatballs; 2 (1/2 cup)	3.0
beans; 1 cup	3.0
yogurt, lowfat; 1 cup	2.6
sweet 'n sour pork; 1.5 cups	2.5
corned beef; 3 ounces	2.5
stew; 1 cup	2.4
chicken liver; 2.5 ounces	2.4
liverwurst; 1 ounce	2.2
lobster; 3.5 ounces (1/2 cup)	2.1
shrimp; 3 ounces	1.7
chicken thigh; 2 ounces	1.6
pork roast; 3 ounces	1.5

Magnesium

Food; Amount	Mg. Magnesium
Bran Buds; 1 cup	240
chick peas (garbanzos); 1 cup	240
soy beans; 1 cup	160
tofu; 1/2 cup	130
Country Morning; 1 cup	120
spinach, cooked; 1 cup	120
All Bran; 1 ounce (1/3 cup)	120
clams; 1/2 cup	115
Instant Breakfast; 1 cup	115
lima beans; 1 cup	110
wheat germ; 1/4 cup	90

FOOD SOURCES OF KEY NUTRIENTS—*Continued*

Magnesium

Food; Amount	Mg. Magnesium
Swiss chard; 1 cup	90
cashews; 1 ounce (15 nuts)	80
buritto; 1	78
beans; 1 cup	74
Bran Chex; 1 cup	72
Buc Wheats; 1 cup	72
refried beans; 1 cup	70
Shredded Wheat; 1 cup	65
chili; 1 cup	65
Brazil nuts; 1 ounce (6 nuts)	65
avocado; 1/2 piece (1/2 cup)	55
banana; 1	55

Iron

Food; Amount	Mg. Iron
prune juice; 1 cup	10.5
oysters; 6	7.6
beef liver; 3 ounces	7.5
lima beans; 1 cup	5.9
baked beans; 1 cup	5.9
beans; 1 cup	4.9
dried peaches; 1/2 cup	4.8
kidney beans; 1 cup	4.6
pork 'n beans; 1 cup	4.6
split peas; 1 cup	4.2
green peas; 1 cup	4.2
asparagus; 1 cup	4.1
spinach, cooked; 1 cup	4.0
clams; 3 ounces	3.5
black-eyed peas; 1 cup	3.2
heel of round, roast; 3 ounces	3.2
blackstrap molasses; 1 tablespoon	3.2
hamburger, lean; 3 ounces	3.0
round steak; 3 ounces	3.0
yellow beans; 1 cup	2.9
green beans; 1 cup	2.9
veal roast; 3 ounces	2.9
pot roast; 3 ounces	2.9
green peas; 1 cup	2.9
veal cutlet; 3 ounces	2.7
hamburger, regular; 3 ounces	2.7
roast pork; 3 ounces	2.7
shrimp; 3 ounces	2.6
pork chop; 3 ounces	2.5

Folic Acid

Food; Amount	Mcg. Folic Acid
asparagus; 1 cup	120
spinach; 1 cup	120

FOOD SOURCES OF KEY NUTRIENTS—*Continued*

Folic Acid

Food; Amount	Mcg. Folic Acid
honeydew melon; 1/4 melon	100
cantaloupe; 1/2 melon	100
orange juice; 1 cup	87
wheat germ; 1 ounce	80
beef liver; 3 ounces	70
beets; 1 cup	60
collards; 1 cup	50
beer; 12 ounces	50
orange; 1 medium	45
turnip greens; 1 cup	40
avocado; 1/2 (1/2 cup)	40
soybeans; 1 cup	40
chef's salad; 2 cups	40
broccoli; 1 cup	40
leeks; 1 cup	40
split peas; 1 cup	40
tangerine; 1 medium	35
tossed salad; 1¼ cups	30
lettuce; 1 cup	30
cauliflower, raw; 1 cup	30
yogurt, lowfat; 1 cup	25
tomato, 1 medium	25
egg; 1	25
banana; 1 medium	25
sesame seeds; 1/4 cup	25

Sodium

Food; Amount	Mg. Sodium
submarine sandwich; 2 cups	3528
kelp; 1 cup	3007
salt; 1 tsp.	2132
dill pickle; 1	1930
veal parmigiani; 1 cup	1825
sauerkraut; 1 cup	1760
chili; 1 cup	1355
potato salad; 1 cup	1300
Tuna Helper; 1 cup	1254
TV dinner—meat loaf; 1	1225
TV dinner—Salisbury steak; 1	1213
Quarter Pounder with cheese; 1	1206
TV dinner—turkey; 1	1200
hash; 1 cup	1190
pork 'n beans; 1 cup	1180
lasagna; 1 cup	1100
macaroni and cheese; 1 cup	1085
TV dinner—chicken; 1	1075
cream soups, canned; 1 cup	1070
ravioli; 1 cup	1065

FOOD SOURCES OF KEY NUTRIENTS—*Continued*

Sodium

Food; Amount	Mg. Sodium
Whopper; 1	1060
vegetable-beef soup; 1 cup	1050
buritto; 1	1047
beefaroni; 1 cup	1044
spaghetti with meat balls; 1 cup	1035
bean soup; 1 cup	1010
beef pot pie; 1.5 cups	1008
egg foo yung; 1 cup	1006
tomato soup; 1 cup	970
spaghetti with sauce; 1¼ cups	955
split pea soup; 1 cup	940
clam chowder; canned; 1 cup	940
TV dinner—beef; 1	938
Big Mac; 1	936
goulash; 1 cup	920
Egg McMuffin; 1	911
Whaler; 1	896
tuna; 3 ounces	865
turkey pot pie; 1.5 cups	864
crab; 1/2 cup (3.5 ounces)	850
chicken pot pie; 1.5 cups	826
TV dinner—pork; 1	821
bouillon; 1 cup	780
chow mein; 1 cup	725
gravy; 1/4 cup	720
onion soup; 1 cup	690
brown rice; 1 cup	685
egg roll; 1 roll	670
ham; 3 ounces	635
pretzels; 10	500
Oat Flakes; 1 cup	500
stuffing; 1/2 cup	497
knockwurst; 3.5 ounces	483
hot dog; 1	477
green olives; 5	465
cottage cheese; 1/2 cup	455
American cheese; 1 ounce	405
luncheon meat; 1 ounce	350

Temperature Chart for Food Safety

"When in doubt, throw the food out"

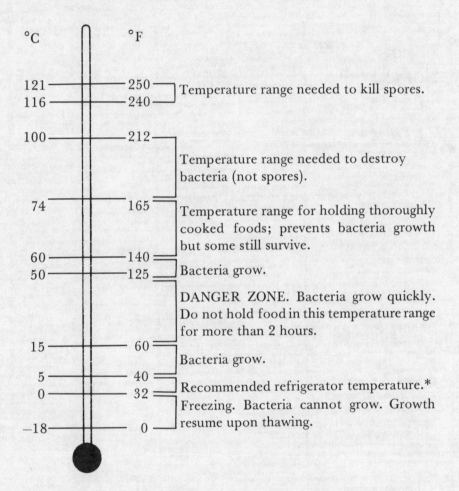

°C   °F

121 ———————— 250 ┐ Temperature range needed to kill spores.
116 ———————— 240 ┘

100 ———————— 212 ┐
                  Temperature range needed to destroy
                  bacteria (not spores).

74 ————————— 165 ┐ Temperature range for holding thoroughly
                  cooked foods; prevents bacteria growth
                  but some still survive.

60 ————————— 140 ┤ Bacteria grow.
50 ————————— 125 ┤

                  DANGER ZONE. Bacteria grow quickly.
                  Do not hold food in this temperature range
                  for more than 2 hours.

15 ————————— 60 ┤ Bacteria grow.

5 —————————— 40 ┤ Recommended refrigerator temperature.*
0 —————————— 32 ┤ Freezing. Bacteria cannot grow. Growth
                 resume upon thawing.
−18 ———————— 0 ┘

Source: Adapted from Temperature Guide to Food Safety. Food and Nutrition Notes, U.S.D.A., No. 25, June 20, 1977.
*Store raw meats for no more than five days and poultry, fish, and ground meat for no more than two days at refrigerator temperature.

CONVERTING COMMON HOUSEHOLD MEASUREMENTS INTO METRIC UNITS

Household Measure	Fluid Ounces (fl. oz.)	Metric Equivalent (ml.)
1 cup (C)	8	240
1 Tablespoon (T)	1/2	15
1 teaspoon (t)	1/6	5
1 gallon (gal)	128	3840
1 quart (qt)	32	960
1 pint (pt)	16	480

Weight	Volume
1 pound = 0.45 kilograms (kg)	1 C = 16 Tbsp.
1 ounce = 28 grams (gm)	1 gallon = 16 cups
	1 qt = 4 C
	1 pt = 2 C

WHERE TO GET MORE INFORMATION ABOUT FOOD AND NUTRITION PROGRAMS

Food Stamps
Food and Nutrition Service
U.S. Department of Agriculture
Washington, D.C. 20250

Special Supplemental Food Program for Women, Infants and Children (WIC)
Supplemental Food Programs
Food and Nutrition Service
U.S. Department of Agriculture
Washington, D.C. 20205
(Or contact your State Health Department.)

Food Safety
Consumer Inquiry Section
Food & Drug Administration
5600 Fishers Lane
Rockville, MD 20852

School Lunch Program
Child Nutrition Programs
Food and Nutrition Service
U.S. Department of Agriculture
Washington, D.C.
(Or contact the Food and Nutrition Service of your state's Department of Education.)

Books on Nutrition

BOOKS ON NUTRITION
HIGHLY RECOMMENDED FOR READERS

General and Family Nutrition

Everybody: A Nutritional Guide to Life. Llewellyn-Jones, D. 1980. Oxford University Press, 200 Madison Avenue, New York, NY. 249 pages.

Realities of Nutrition. Deutsch, R. D. 1976. Bull Publishing Co., Palo Alto, CA. 405 pages.

A Diet for Living. Mayer, J. 1975. David McKay Co., Inc. Orangeburg, NY. 293 pages.

Dietary Guidelines, "Nutrition and Your Health." Pamphlet available from Consumer Information Center, Pueblo, CA, 81009. Single copy free. Refer to publication no. 565#.

Your Money's Worth in Foods, Home and Garden Bulletin No. 183, revised in 1979. Science and Education Administration, USDA, Washington, D.C. 20250. 29 pages. Single copy free.

The American Diabetes Association. American Dietetic Association Family Cookbook. 1980. Prentice-Hall, Inc., Englewood Cliffs, NJ. 391 pages.

The Family Health Cookbook. White, A. and the Society for Nutrition Education. 1980. David McKay Co., Inc., Orangeburg, NY. 284 pages.

Eat Well, Be Well. Jane Brody's Nutrition Book, Brody, J. W. W. Norton & Co., New York, NY. 552 pages.

Vegetarian Diets

Cooking with Low-Cost Proteins. Clamp, B. D. 1976. Acro Publishing, New York, NY.

Laurel's Kitchen: A Handbook for Vegetarian Cookery and Nutrition. Robertson, L. and others. 1976. Nilgiri Press, Petaluma, CA. 500 pages.

Diet for a Small Planet. Lappe, F. M. 1971. Friends fo the Earth/Ballentine Books, Inc. New York, NY. 432 pages.

Breast-Feeding

Breast Feeding, U.S. DHEW, 1979. Bureau of Community Health Services, Health Services Administration, Public Health Service, 5600 Fishers Lane, Rockville, MD. 20857. DHEW publication no. (HSA) 79-5102. 22 pages. Single copy free.

Nursing Your Baby. Pryor, K. 1973. Harper and Row, Publishers. New York, NY. 304 pages.

Breast-Feeding: A Practical Guide for the Medical Profession. Lawrence, R. D. 1980. C. V. Mosby Co., St. Louis, MO.

Infant Feeding and Nutrition

No-Nonsense Nutrition: For Your Baby's First Year. Heslin, J. and others. 1978. CBI Publishing Co., Boston, Mass. 284 pages.

Child Nutrition

What's to Eat? And Other Questions Kids Ask about Food. USDA Yearbook 1979. 1980. Government Printing Office, Washington, D.C. 20402. 42 pages.

Food, Nutrition, and the Young Child. Endreas, J. B. and Rockwell, R. D. 1980. C. V. Mosby Co., Inc., St. Louis, MO. 312 pages.

SOME SOURCES CONSULTED BY THE AUTHOR

History of Diet and Pregnancy

Antonov, A.N. Children born during the siege of Leningrad in 1942. *Journal of Pediatrics* 30(3):250-259, 1947.

Becker, J.E., Bickerstaff, H.J., and Eastman, N.J. Nutrition in relation to pregnancy and lactation. *American Journal of Public Health* 31(12):1263-1270, 1941.

Bingham, A.W. The prevention of obstetric complications by diet and exercise. *American Journal of Obstetrics and Gynecology* 23(1):38-44, 1932.

Davis, C.H. Weight in pregnancy: Its value as a routine test. *American Journal of Obstetrics and Gynecology* 6(5):575-581, 1923.

Dieckmann, W.J., Turner, D.F., and Ruby, B.A. Diet regulation and controlled weight in pregnancy. *American Journal of Obstetrics and Gynecology* 50(6):701-712, 1945.

Fairbairn, J.S. *A Textbook for Midwives*. London: Oxford University Press, 1914.

Guillemeau. *Childbirth*. London, 1612.

Jellet, H., and Madill, D.G. *A Manual of Midwifery*. 4th ed. New York: Wood, 1929.

Johnstone, R.W. *A Textbook of Midwifery*. 11th ed. London: Adam and Charles Black, 1942.

Klein, J. The relationship of maternal weight gain to the weight of the newborn infant. *American Journal of Obstetrics and Gynecology* 52(4):574-580, 1946.

Lush, W.T. *The Science and Art of Midwifery*. New York: Appleton, 1885.

Reed, C.B., and Cooley, B.I. *A Textbook of Obstetrics*. St. Louis: Mosby, 1939.

Reynolds, E. *Practical Midwifery, A Handbook of Treatment*. New York: Wood, 1892.

Smith, C.A. Effects of maternal malnutrition upon the newborn infant in Holland, 1944-45. *Journal of Pediatrics* 30(3):229-243, 1947.

Smith, G.F.D. Effects of the state of nutrition of the mother during pregnancy and labour on the condition of the child at birth and for the first few days of life. *The Lancet* 2(4845):54-56, July 8, 1916.

Stein, Z., et al. *Famine and Human Development: The Dutch Hunger Winter of 1944-45*. London: Oxford University Press, 1975.

Nutrition and the Course and Outcome of Pregnancy

Beal, V.A. Nutritional studies during pregnancy. 2. Dietary intake, maternal weight gain, and size of infant. *Journal of the American Dietetic Association* 58(4):321-326, 1971.

Berger, L. and Susser, M.W. Low-birth weight and prenatal nutrition: An interpretive review. *Pediatrics* 46(6):946-966, 1970.

Brown, J.E., and Toma, R. Food cravings experienced by women during normal pregnancies. In preparation, 1981.

Burke, B.S. et al. Nutrition studies during pregnancy. 4. Relation of protein content of mother's diet during pregnancy to birth length, birth weight, and condition of the infant. *Journal of Pediatrics* 23(5):506-515, 1943.

Chase, H.C. The position of the United States in international comparisons of health status. *American Journal of Public Health* 62(4):581-589, 1972.

Chesley, L.C. *Hypertension disorders of pregnancy*. New York: Appleton-Century Crofts, 1978.

Ebbs, J.H., et al. The influence of prenatal diet on the mother and child. *Milbank Memorial Fund Quarterly* 20(1):35-46, 1942.

Fleming, A.F., et al. Anaemia during pregnancy. *The Lancet* 1(7900):225, January 25, 1975.

Higgens, A.C. Nutritional status and the outcome of pregnancy. *Journal of the Canadian Dietetic Association* 37:17-36, 1976.

Jacobson, H.N. Current concepts in nutrition. Diet in pregnancy. *New England Journal of Medicine* 297(19):1051-1053, 1977.

Jukes, T.H. Food additives. *New England Journal of Medicine*, 297(8):427-430, 1977.

Kaminski, M., Goujard, J., and Rumeau-Rouquette, C. Prediction of low birth weight and prematurity by a multiple regression analysis with maternal characteristics known since the beginning of the pregnancy. *International Journal of Epidemiology* 2(2):195-204, 1973.

King, J.C. Protein metabolism during pregnancy. *Clinics in Perinatology* 2(2):243-254, 1975.

Latham, M.C. and Cobos, F. The effects of malnutrition on intellectual development and learning. *American Journal of Public Health* 61(7):1307-1325, 1971.

Lechtig, A., et al. Influence of maternal nutrition on birth weight. *American Journal of Clinical Nutrition* 28(11):1223-1233, 1975.

Lechtig, A., et al. A simple assessment of the risk of low birth weight to select women for nutritional intervention. *American Journal of Obstetrics and Gynecology* 125(1):25-34, 1976.

Maternal Nutrition and the Course of Pregnancy. Committee on Maternal Nutrition, Food and Nutrition Board, National Academy of Sciences, National Research Council, Washington, D.C., 1970.

McCarthy, C.P., et al. Alterations in body composition during pregnancy. *American Journal of Obstetrics and Gynecology* 77(5):1038-1053, 1959.

Naeye, R.L. Malnutrition: Probable causes of fetal growth retardation. *Archives of Pathology* 79(March):284-291, 1965.

Naeye, R.L., Blanc, W., and Paul, C. Effects of maternal nutrition on the human fetus. *Pediatrics* 52(4):494-503, 1973.

Niswander, K.R. and Gordon, M. *The Women and Their Pregnancies: The Collaborative Perinatal Study of the National Institute of Neurological Disease and Stroke*. Phil.: W.B. Saunders, 1972.

Osofsky, H.J. Relationships between nutrition during pregnancy and subsequent infant and child development. *Obstetrical and Gynecological Survey* 30(4):227-241, 1975.

Pike, R. and Smiciklas, H. A reappraisal of sodium restriction during pregnancy. *International Journal of Gynaecology and Obstetrics* 10(1):1-8, 1972.

Pitkin, R.M. Vitamins and minerals in pregnancy. *Clinics in Perinatology* 2(2):221-232, 1975.

Primrose, T. and Higgins, Agnes. A study in human antepartum nutrition. *Journal of Reproductive Medicine* 7(6):257-264, 1971.

Sack, R.A. The large infant. *American Journal of Obstetrics and Gynecology* 104(2):195-204, 1969.

Sullivan, J.M. Hypertension in pregnancy. *Clinics in Perinatology* 1(2):369-384, 1974.

Thomson, A.M. Diet in pregnancy. 3. Diet in relation to the course and outcome of pregnancy. *British Journal of Nutrition* 13:509-525, 1959.

Thomson, A.M. and Hytten, F.E., Nutrition during pregnancy. *World Review of Nutrition and Dietetics* 16:22-45, 1973.

Tompkins, W.T., and Wiehl, D.G. Maternal and newborn studies at Philadelphia Lying-In Hospital. Maternal studies: III. Toxemia and maternal nutrition. *Proceedings of the Annual Conference of the Milbank Memorial Fund*, 1954, pp. 62-90.

Lactation

American Academy of Pediatrics. Breast-feeding. *Pediatrics* 62(4):591-601, 1978.

Applebaum, R.M. The modern management of successful breastfeeding. *Pediatric Clinics of North America* 17(1):203-225, 1970.

Archavsky, I.A. Immediate breastfeeding of newborn infant in the prophylaxis of the so-called physiological loss of weight. *Vopr. Pediatr.* 20:45-52, 1953.

Brilliant, L.B., et al. Breast-milk monitoring to measure Michigan's contamination with polybrominated biphenols. *The Lancet* 2(8091):643-646, September 23, 1978.

Lawrence, R.A. *Breastfeeding: A Guide for the Medical Profession*. St. Louis: C.V. Mosby Co., 1980.

MacKeith, R. and Wood, C. *Infant Feeding and Feeding Difficulties*. 4th ed. London, 1971.

Sosa, R., Kennell, J.H., Klaus, M. and Urrutia, J.J. The effect of early mother-infant contact on breast feeding, infection, and growth. In Ciba Foundation Symposium 45 (new series), *Breastfeeding and the Mother*, 45:179-193, 1976.

Worthington-Roberts, B.S., and Taylor, L.E., Guidance for lactating mothers. In *Nutrition in Pregnancy and Lactation*. 2nd ed. St. Louis: C.V. Mosby, 1981.

Alcohol in Pregnancy

Little, R.E. Moderate alcohol use during pregnancy and decreased infant birth weight. *American Journal of Public Health* 67(12):1154-1156, 1977.

Mendelson, J.H. The fetal alcohol syndrome. *New England Journal of Medicine* 299(10):556, 1978.

Research Resources Report, Fetal Alcohol Syndrome. NIH Division of Research Resources, PHS, DHHS, Washington, D.C.

Saccharin

Report of Committee for a Study on Saccharin and Food Safety, National Research Council/National Academy of Sciences. Washington, D.C., 1978.

Pines, W.L. The saccharin ban. *FDA Consumer*. May 1977, pp. 10-13.

Environmental Contaminants in Food

Atkinson, S.A. Chemical contamination of human milk; a review of current knowledge. *Journal of the Canadian Dietetic Association*, 40:223-226, 1979.

Kendrick, E. Testing for environmental contaminants in human milk. *Pediatrics*, 66:470-472, 1980.

Kodama, H. and Ota, H. Transfer of polychlorinated biphenyls to infants from their mothers. *Archives of Environmental Health*, 35:95-100, 1980.

Rogan, W.J., Bagniewska, A., and Damstra, T. Pollutants in breast milk. *New England Journal of Medicine*, 302:1450-1453, 1980.

Wickizer, T.M. and Brilliant, L.B. Testing for polychlorinated biphenyls in human milk. *Pediatrics*, 68:411-415, 1981.

Nutrition Glossary

Abortion: Loss of an embryo or fetus usually within the first three months of pregnancy.

Absorption: The taking up of fluids, gases, and nutrients by the gastrointestinal tract.

Allergy: Unusual or exaggerated sensitivity to a substance that is harmless in similar amounts to most people.

Amino Acids: The chemical building blocks from which proteins are made. Amino acids are classified into two groups: essential and nonessential.

> **Essential:** Amino acids that cannot be produced by the body and must be supplied by the diet. The eight essential amino acids for adults are isoleucine, leucine, lysine, methionine, phenylalanine, theronine, tryptophan, and valine. In addition, histidine and agrinine are required by children for growth.

> **Nonessential:** Amino acids that can be produced by the body provided the diet contains enough nitrogen-containing foods. Nonessential amino acids are alanine, aspartic acid, arginine, citrulline, cystine, glutamic acid, glycine, hydroxyglutamic acid, hydroxyproline, norleucine, proline, serine, and tyrosine.

Anemia: Reduction in size or number of the red blood cells, of the quantity of hemoglobin, or of both, resulting in decreased capacity of the blood to carry oxygen. The symptoms of anemia are varied and include breathlessness on exertion, easy fatigue, pallor, dizziness, insomnia, and lack of appetite. Anemias may be caused by a deficient intake of nutrients necessary for the formation of blood. Iron, protein, folic acid, vitamin B_{12}, and vitamin C deficiencies interefere with blood formation. Anemia may also be due to blood loss, inherited conditions, and other disorders.

Antacids: Substances that neutralize or reduce the acidity of fluids in the digestive tract. Two common antacids are aluminum hydroxide and magnesium oxide.

Appetite: The desire for food, founded on learning or memory and related to the agreeable taste, smell, or appearance of food.

Basal Metabolism: Energy, or calories, used by the body for maintaining processes such as body temperature, circulation, and muscle tone. Basal metabolism increases during pregnancy, primarily because of increases in body weight, circulation, and protein-tissue formation.

Basic Food Groups: Classes of foods listed together under one heading because of their similarities as good sources of certain nutrients. The basic food groups are used in planning and evaluating diets for nutritional adequacy.

Calorie: A unit of heat. In nutrition, calorie refers to the amount of heat a food substance will release when completely burned. Approximately 3500 extra calories from food are needed to produce one pound of body fat. Conversely, reducing food intake by 3500 calories below usual intake will cause a weight loss of one pound.

Carbohydrate: The class of foods that includes simple sugars and starches. Fiber is a carbohydrate, although it is not digested or absorbed by the body. Carbohydrates are the major sources of calories in most diets.

Carcinogen: Cancer-producing agent or substances.

Cardiac: Pertaining to the heart.

Cardiac Output: The quantity of blood pumped into circulation by the heart per minute. Cardiac output increases substantially during pregnancy.

Cholesterol: The chief sterol in the body found in all tissues, especially the brain, nerves, adrenal cortex, and liver. It is also a constituent of bile and serves as a precursor of vitamin D. Cholesterol in the body comes from two sources: dietary cholesterol, chiefly from egg yolk, liver, and meats; and cholesterol made by the liver and other organs. High blood cholesterol levels are related to hardening of the arteries, high blood pressure, stone formation, and other diseases. Blood levels of cholesterol rise substantially during pregnancy.

Constipation: Infrequent or difficult bowel movements. Common causes of constipation include a diet low in fiber and fluids, lack of exercise, excessive use of laxatives, and anxiety or worry.

Convenience Foods: Foods that have been partially or completely prepared to save time in food preparation.

Diabetic Diet: A diet prescribed for a person with diabetes. This diet follows the pattern of a normal diet for maintenance of good health and normal activity. It is no longer necessary to require a diabetic (who is experiencing no complications from diabetes) to follow detailed dietary regulations and precise food measurements and meal patterns. Except for simple sugars that are rapidly absorbed and can produce high blood-sugar peaks, a diabetic can have more freedom in his or her choice of foods. However, individualization is the rule. The dietary requirements of diabetics differ with the type and extent of insulin received and the amount of activity performed. The most important consideration is adjustment of total caloric intake to attain and maintain desirable body weight. Also important are the proper spacing and regularity of meals, particularly among those receiving insulin, to avoid low blood-sugar levels.

Diarrhea: The frequent passage of loose and watery stools. Severe or prolonged diarrhea can lead to dehydration and mineral losses from the body.

Diet: The foods and beverages a person eats on a regular basis. The diet of most adult Americans includes 200 to 350 different foods and beverages out of around 3500 types of foods and beverages available.

Diet, Balanced: A diet containing all the required nutrients in proper proportion with respect to one another for optimum nutrition.

Dietary Counseling: A process of providing individualized professional guidance to assist a person in adjusting his or her daily food consumption to meet health needs.

Dietetics: The science of the use of foods in health and disease.

Dietitian: One who is professionally qualified by education and experience to provide nutritional care, and apply the science and art of nutrition in helping people of all ages, sick or well, individually or in groups, to meet their nutritional needs. The American Dietetic Association is responsible for qualifications and registration of dietitians in the United States.

Digestion: The mechanical and chemical breakdown of food substances into constituent parts. The conversion of food into smaller and simpler units that can be absorbed by the body.

Eclampsia: A condition usually occurring during the latter half of pregnancy characterized by edema, high blood pressure, proteinuria, and convulsions. The condition is referred to as preeclampsia in the absence of convulsions. Both terms, eclampsia and preeclampsia, are collectively called toxemia of pregnancy.

Edema: A condition in which the body tissues contain an excessive amount of fluid. The swelling of body tissues from the excess fluid may be throughout the body or in the legs and ankles, depending upon the seriousness of the condition.

Embryo: The developing human organism from conception to eight weeks in the uterus.

"Empty Calorie" Foods: A term used to describe foods and beverages that are high in calories and contain small amounts of nutrients. Some nutritionists and mothers have been heard to call such products "junk food."

Energy: Capacity to do work. Energy needed by the body for movement and body processes is obtained from food. The energy available from foods is released for use by the body when foods are broken down by enzymes. The amount of energy available from foods is measured in terms of calories.

Energy Balance: (Also called calorie balance.) The equilibrium between calorie intake and calorie output. When more calories are available from foods eaten than are needed by the body, the surplus is stored as fat. When fewer calories are consumed than needed, the body draws upon the fat stores.

Enrichment: The addition of vitamins and minerals (specifically, thiamin, riboflavin, niacin, and iron) to processed cereal and grain products to restore the amount lost in milling and processing.

Estrogen: The name given to the female sex hormones produced by the ovary. Estrogens include estrone, estradial, and esterone. Estrogens are responsible for the development of physical sexual characteristics and have a profound influence on reproduction, how the body uses nutrients, and many other processes.

Fetus: The baby within the uterus from the third month of pregnancy until birth. Before three months, the term ebryo is used.

Fiber: Substances, primarily carbohydrates, that are found in foods but that are not digested by the body. Fiber is needed to promote regular bowel movements. Whole grain breads and cereals, legumes, nuts, seeds, and fruits and vegetables are good sources of dietary fiber.

Food Additive: Substances that have been added to food, either intentionally or unintentionally, that are not normally part of the food. Food additives are used to improve the nutritional value, appearance, shelf-life, texture, and flavor of foods. Some additives unintentionally end up in food through processing, production, storage, and packaging. Accidental contaminants, such as mercury or lead, are not considered food additives.

Food Poisoning: Toxic condition caused by eating a food contaminated with bacteria. Refer to the "Temperature Chart for Food Safety" given on page 107 for a guide to preventing food poisoning.

Fortification: Addition of one or more nutrients such as vitamins, minerals, amino acids, and protein concentrates to food so that it contains more nutrients than were originally present. For example, the addition of vitamin A to margarine, vitamin D to milk, lysine to bread, and iodine to salt.

Gastrointestinal Tract: Refers to the whole of the digestive tract from the mouth through the stomach, intestines, and anus.

Gestation: Pregnancy; the period of fetal development.

Gestational Age: The age of a fetus or newborn computed from the first day of the last menstrual period to birth. Most babies are born within a gestational period of thirty-eight to forty-two weeks. Babies that are born unusually small considering the length of pregnancy, or gestation, are classified as small-for-gestational age. Babies that are unusually large for the length of the pregnancy are classified as large-for-gestational age.

Glucose Tolerance Test (GTT): The test that measures the ability of the body to use a certain amount of glucose. It is performed after a twelve-hour fast. The person is given 50 to 100 g. of glucose. Blood samples for a glucose analysis are obtained before the glucose is taken and then one-half, one, two, three, and four hours after ingestion. A normal individual shows a rise in blood sugar about one-half hour after ingestion of glucose, but the blood-sugar level returns to normal after two hours. A person with diabetes shows a much higher rise in blood sugar after one-half hour, which continues to rise even higher after two hours and remains higher than normal after four hours.

Health: State of physical, mental, and emotional well-being, not merely the freedom from disease or the absence of any ailment.

Hearburn: A burning sensation felt in the esophagus when acidic fluids are forced up from the stomach. It may occur ten to fifteen minutes after eating a big meal, especially if a person lies down after the meal. During pregnancy, heartburn usually results from the pressure of the baby on the stomach.

Hematocrit: A laboratory test that determines the volume of red blood cells in a certain amount of blood. The hematocrit result is used to test for iron deficiency anemia during pregnancy. A hematocrit of less than 33 percent may indicate the development of anemia.

Hemoglobin: The iron-containing substance in red blood cells. Hemoglobin carries the oxygen from the lungs to the tissues. A test for hemoglobin level is usually done several times during pregnancy. A hemoglobin level of less than 11 g. percent is suggestive of iron deficiency anemia.

Hemorrhoid: An enlarged bundle of vessels located around the anus.

Heredity: The tendency of a human to reproduce the characteristics of his or her ancestors. Characteristics of heredity are carried in genes located within the sperm cell and ovum.

Hormone: A chemical substance produced by the body that is carried in the bloodstream to other parts of the body. Each hormone has a specific effect on only those cells and tissues that serve as "targets" for hormonal action.

Hunger: A physical sensation resulting from the lack of food and a sign that food is needed by the body. Hunger is usually accompanied by weakness and an overwhelming desire to eat. It is different from appetite, which is a pleasant sensation based on enjoyment of foods and eating, and not necessarily on the need for food.

Hypertension: An increase in blood pressure above normal. Blood pressure varies considerably among individuals. Hypertension often causes dizziness, headaches, poor vision, shortness of breath, chest pain, and poor memory. Blood pressure normally decreases during the early part of pregnancy but returns to pre-pregnancy levels toward the end of pregnancy.

Immunity: Resistance to a particular disease. Immunity may be received by the fetus from the mother's blood or may occur as a result of having a disease or receiving a vaccination.

Incidence: The number of new cases of a disease or disorder appearing in a set amount of time (usually one year) within a population.

Infant: Babies up to one year of age.

Infant Formula: A breastmilk substitute prepared for infants according to a specific formula.

Infection: The transfer of disease from one person to another by a variety of routes.

Lactation: Breast-feeding. The production of milk by the breast. The amount of milk a woman produces is affected by her nutritional status, the frequency and length of sucking by the baby, certain drugs (particularly birth-control pills), and hormones.

Lactose Intolerance: Failure to digest lactose, a primary component of milk owing to the lack of the enzyme lactose which digests it. Lactose intolerance among infants results in failure to grow and diarrhea if human or cow's milk is given. The condition is extremely rare among infants, particularly breast-fed infants. Adults not used to drinking milk may develop gas pains and diarrhea after drinking a sizable amount of milk. In these cases, small amounts of milk should be taken until the body can produce enough lactase to properly digest it.

Legumes: Edible seeds, such as beans, peas, peanuts, and soybeans.

Low Birth-Weight Infant: An infant who weighs less than five pounds, eight ounces, or 2500 g. at birth.

Malformation: A deformity or defective formation of some body part or parts.

Malnutrition: A state of poor health with symptoms that can be identified as the result of an inadequate or excessive intake of one or more essential nutrients.

Menarche: The beginning of menstrual periods.

Menstruation: The periodic cycle, usually twenty-eight to thirty days, characterized by uterine bleeding or menstrual flow. It is peculiar to women from puberty to menopause. It normally lasts from three to seven days with a bloody discharge of about one-half cup in total.

Nutrient: A substance needed by the body to perform one or more of the following functions: to provide energy, to build and repair tissues, and to regulate life processes. The body uses about sixty different nutrients from foods. Nutrients are grouped into six categories; proteins, fats, carbohydrates, vitamins, minerals, and water. All nutrients are needed for growth and health. No one nutrient is more important than any other.

Nutrient Deficiency Disease: A disease or disorder caused by a dietary deficiency of one or more nutrients. The disease or disorder can be prevented by eating an adequate diet, or in most cases cured by supplying the deficient nutrient or nutrients.

Nutrient Toxicity: A disease or disorder caused by taking an excessive amount of certain vitamin and mineral supplements.

Nutrition: The science of how the body uses foods and how foods influence health and disease.

Nutritional Status: The health condition of a person as influenced by the consumption and utilization of foods.

Nutritionist: A dietitian with graduate-level training in nutrition who applies the science of nutrition to improving health, the prevention of disease, and the treatment of disease.

Obesity: A condition that exists when a person's weight exceeds by 20 percent the average weight for persons of the same sex, height, and age.

Overweight: A condition that exists when a person's weight exceeds by ten to twenty percent the average weight for persons of the same sex, height, and age.

Pica: The craving and eating of materials not considered food. Common substances craved and consumed include clay, dirt, laundry starch, and ice. Pica may develop during pregnancy and be abandoned after delivery.

Preeclampsia: A condition of pregnancy characterized by hypertension, proteinuria, and swelling. The signs of preeclampsia may not be noted until after mid-pregnancy. However, the condition itself begins to develop earlier in pregnancy.

Pregnancy: Also called gestation; the condition of having a developing embryo or fetus in the body after the union of an ovum and a spermatozoan. In women the period of pregnancy is about 266 to 280 days. It is divided into three main phases: implantation, the first two weeks of gestation during which the fertilized ovum becomes embedded in the wall of the uterus and the placenta develops; organogenesis, the next ten weeks during which the developing fetal tissue undergoes organ formation; and growth, the remaining six months, characterized by a rapid growth in organ size and body weight.

Premature: A baby born before thirty-seven weeks of gestation. In the past, the term was applied to low birth-weight infants (less than five-and-one-half pounds). The term is now used solely to indicate a shorter-than-average gestational period.

Protein: The source of amino acids needed from foods. Protein is a structural component of all tissues. An important function of protein is the manufacture of body tissues such as muscles, bones, nerves, teeth, hair, skin, blood, and organs. All enzymes and some hormones are composed of protein.

Protein Quality: An attribute of a protein that depends on the kinds and amounts of amino acids present. In general, plant proteins are lacking or "limiting" in the essential amino acids lysine, methionine, thereonine, and tryptophan. Animal proteins are of high quality, or are said to be complete proteins. A complete protein contains all the essential amino acids in amounts sufficient for growth and life maintenance. An incomplete protein cannot support life or growth. Incomplete sources of protein can be used effectively for growth and repair by combining them with small amounts of complete proteins, or by mixing several plant proteins to obtain a complete assortment of amino acids in the amounts needed for growth and repair.

Proteinuria: The presence of protein or amino acids in urine.

Recommended Dietary Allowances: The specific term used by the Food and Nutrition Board of the National Research Council of the National Academy of Sciences (NAS/NRC) for recommendations for daily intake of specific nutrients for groups of healthy individuals according to age and sex. The recommended dietary allowances (RDA), designed to be adequate for practically all the population of the United States, allow for a margin of safety.

Satiety: The lack of desire to continue to eat. A feeling of satisfaction after eating.

Starvation: Complete or partial absence from food for varying lengths of time.

Stress: Emotional or physical events that affect normal body functions and nutrient needs. There are several types of stress that affect nutritional status.

> *Physical Stress:* Heavy labor, physical exertion, or strenuous exercise may place stress on the individual and increase the body's requirement for calories and certain other nutrients.

> *Physiological Stress:* Increased nutrient demands placed upon a person such as occur in fever, infection, chronic illness, surgery, pregnancy, or lactation.

> *Psychological Stress:* Emotional factors that affect appetite, digestion, and the way the body uses nutrients.

Toxicity: A pathological condition that results when harmful substances are ingested or when excessive amounts of normally harmless substances are ingested.

Undernutrition: Inadequate intake of one or more nutrients and/or of calories.

Underweight: The term applied to individuals whose body weights are more than 10 percent below average for individuals of the same age, sex, and height.

Uterus: The womb. A pear-shaped, hollow muscular organ in the female that shelters and nourishes the fetus during pregnancy. Except during pregnancy, the uterus is about three inches long, two inches wide, and one inch thick. It includes the fundus (the upper and broad portion), the body (the central part), and the cervix at the bottom.

Vegans: Individuals who eat only food and food products from plant sources; all animal foods including meat, fish, poultry, milk, eggs, cheese, and seafoods in any form are avoided.

Vegetarians: Those who refrain from eating meat of any kind, but use milk, milk products, and eggs; these people are more specifically described as ovo-lacto-vegetarians. Those who refrain from eating meat and eggs are called lactovegetarians.

Vulnerability: Susceptibility to injury. In nutrition, the phrase vulnerable group refers to infants, children, pregnant or lactating women, and elderly people—groups particularly prone to develop nutritional disorders.

Water Balance: Balance between water input and output. Water intake comes from fluids and beverages, as part of food, or as a product of the breakdown of foods in the body. The channels of water output are through the kidneys (urine), the skin (sweat and insensible perspiration), the lungs (expired air), and the gastrointestinal tract (saliva and feces). Water intake must equal output; a difference results in edema or dehydration, depending on whether intake is greater or less than output. Control of water intake is by thirst. Water output is controlled by hormones. Abnormal losses of water may occur in diarrhea, excessive vomiting, and severe burns.

Weaning: The period from the first consistent addition of a semi-solid or solid food into the infant diet.

My Diet

Date_____

Time of Day	What I Ate and Drank	Amount Consumed
Morning		
Mid-morning		
Noon		
Afternoon		
Evening		
Late evening		

My Diet

Time of Day	What I Ate and Drank	Date_____ Amount Consumed
Morning		
Mid-morning		
Noon		
Afternoon		
Evening		
Late evening		

My Diet

Time of Day	What I Ate and Drank	Date_____ Amount Consumed
Morning		
Mid-morning		
Noon		
Afternoon		
Evening		
Late evening		

My Diet

Date _____

Time of Day	What I Ate and Drank	Amount Consumed
Morning		
Mid-morning		
Noon		
Afternoon		
Evening		
Late evening		

My Diet

Time of Day	What I Ate and Drank	Date_____ Amount Consumed
Morning		
Mid-morning		
Noon		
Afternoon		
Evening		
Late evening		

My Diet

Time of Day	What I Ate and Drank	Date_____ Amount Consumed
Morning		
Mid-morning		
Noon		
Afternoon		
Evening		
Late evening		

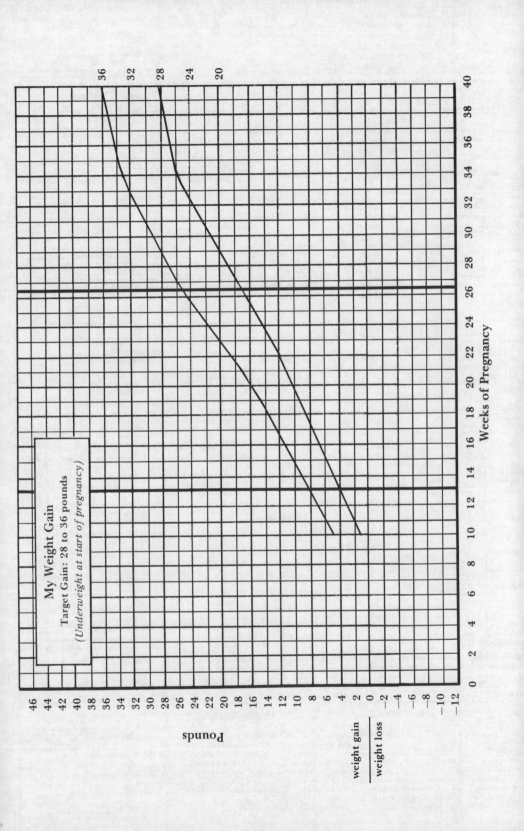

My Weight Gain

Target Gain: 28 to 36 pounds

(Underweight at start of pregnancy)

Weeks of Pregnancy

Pounds

weight gain
weight loss

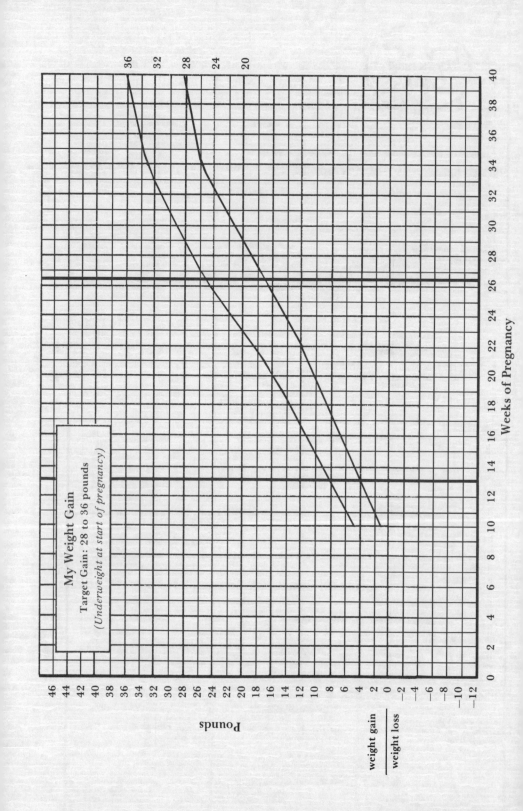

My Weight Gain

Target Gain: 28 to 36 pounds
(Underweight at start of pregnancy)

Weeks of Pregnancy

Pounds

weight gain
—————
weight loss

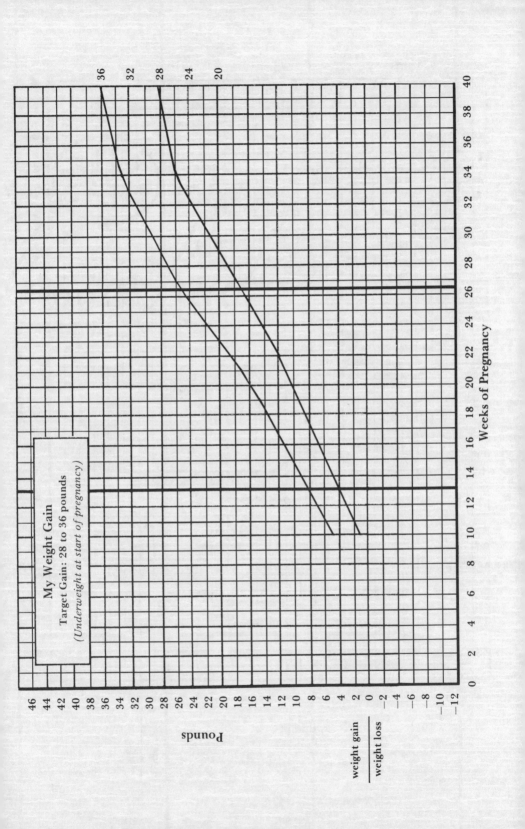

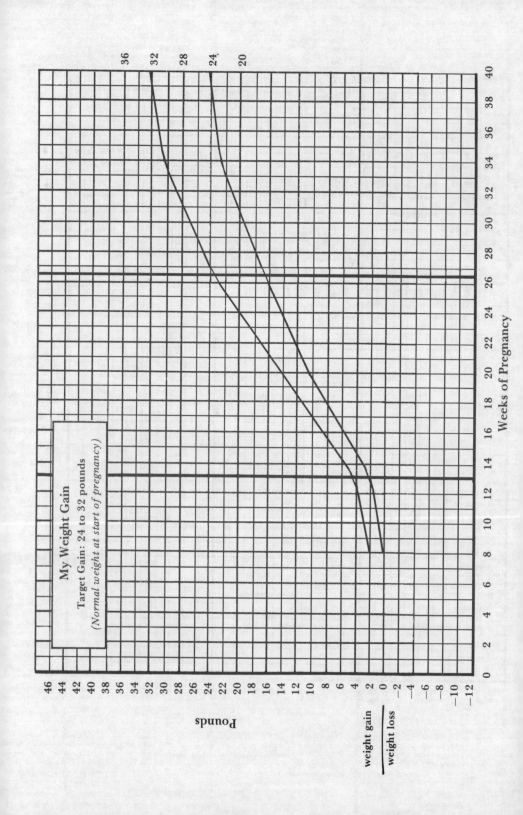

My Weight Gain

Target Gain: 24 to 32 pounds
(Normal weight at start of pregnancy)

Weeks of Pregnancy

Pounds

weight gain
weight loss

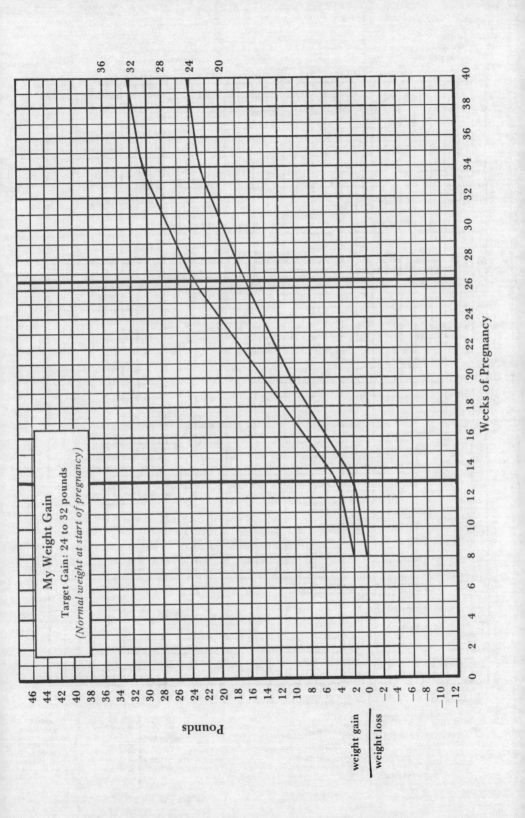

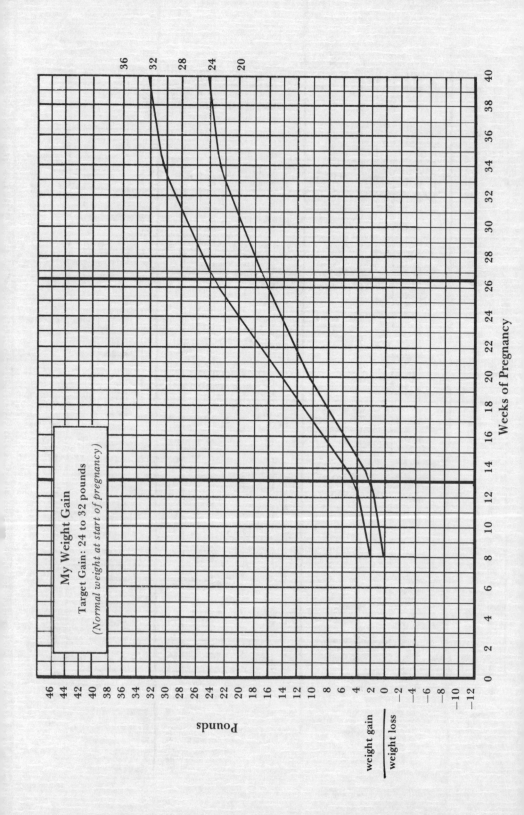

My Weight Gain

Target Gain: 24 to 32 pounds

(Normal weight at start of pregnancy)

Pounds

46
44
42
40
38
36
34
32
30
28
26
24
22
20
18
16
14
12
10
8
6
4
2
0
−2
−4
−6
−8
−10
−12

weight gain

weight loss

36
32
28
24
20

Weeks of Pregnancy

0 2 4 6 8 10 12 14 16 18 20 22 24 26 28 30 32 34 36 38 40

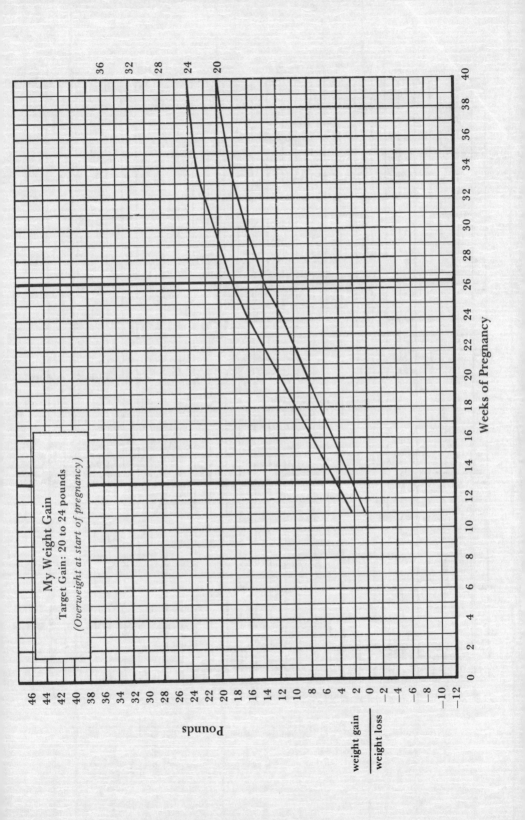

My Weight Gain
Target Gain: 20 to 24 pounds
(Overweight at start of pregnancy)

Pounds

weight gain
weight loss

Weeks of Pregnancy

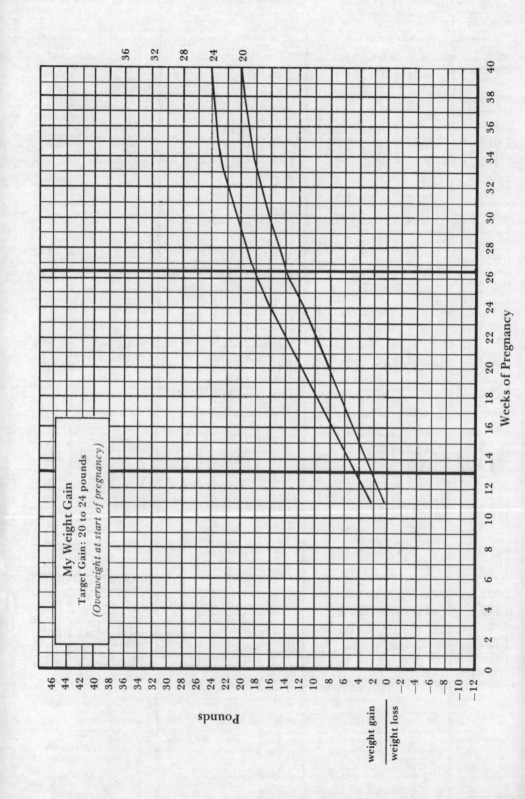

My Weight Gain

Target Gain: 20 to 24 pounds

(Overweight at start of pregnancy)

Pounds

46 44 42 40 38 36 34 32 30 28 26 24 22 20 18 16 14 12 10 8 6 4 2 0
weight gain
─────────
weight loss
-2 -4 -6 -8 -10 -12

Weeks of Pregnancy

0 2 4 6 8 10 12 14 16 18 20 22 24 26 28 30 32 34 36 38 40

36 32 28 24 20

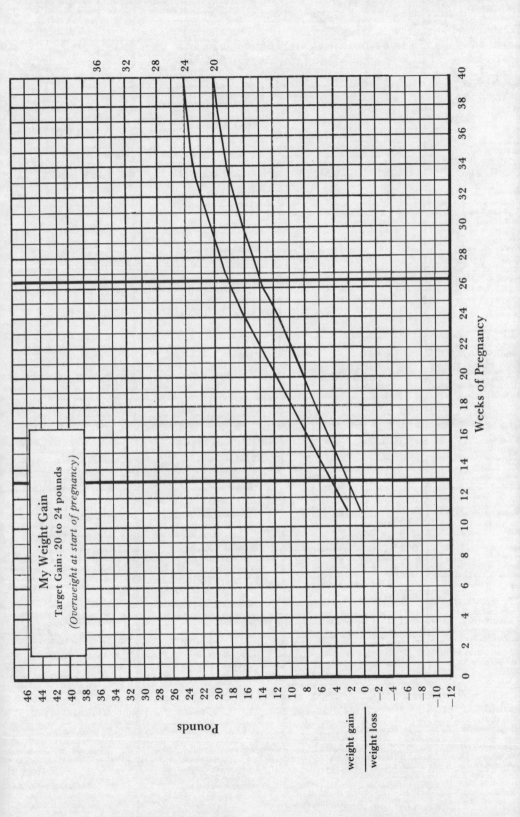

My Weight Gain
Target Gain: 20 to 24 pounds
(Overweight at start of pregnancy)

Pounds

weight gain
—————————
weight loss

Weeks of Pregnancy

Index

Judith E. Brown is a registered dietician with a masters degree in public health from the University of Michigan and a doctorate in human nutrition from Florida State University. She is director of the program in public health nutrition at the University of Minnesota, where she teaches maternal and child nutrition to nurses, nurse-midwives, and physicians. Brown is an elected member of the American Institute of Nutrition.